OVERCOMING RESISTANCE TO CANCER IMMUNOTHERAPY

Unleashing Resilience for Effective Treatment

Dr. Bhratri Bhushan
MBBS, MD, DM

Copyright © 2023 Dr. Bhratri Bhushan

CONTENTS

PREFACE

Cancer immunotherapy has emerged as a transformative paradigm in the field of oncology, offering unprecedented advancements and renewed hope in the treatment of various malignancies. By harnessing the innate power of the immune system to recognize and eliminate cancer cells, immunotherapy has demonstrated remarkable efficacy and durable responses in a subset of patients. However, a formidable challenge that has surfaced is the development of resistance to immunotherapy, which significantly limits its effectiveness and hampers the realization of its full potential.

This book is a comprehensive exploration of the intricate mechanisms underlying cancer immunotherapy resistance and an in-depth examination of the strategies being developed to overcome this formidable obstacle. It represents the culmination of extensive research, collaborative endeavors, and the collective dedication of scientists, clinicians, and researchers committed to unraveling the complexities surrounding immunotherapy resistance.

Within the pages of this book, we embark on a profound journey to comprehend the multifaceted factors that contribute to resistance. We delve into the intricate interplay between the tumor and the immune system, investigating the immunological, genetic, and microenvironmental dynamics that shape treatment responses. We meticulously examine the alterations in antigen presentation machinery, the upregulation of immune checkpoint molecules, the presence of inhibitory immune cells, the secretion of immunosuppressive factors, and the emergence of resistant tumor cell clones, among other critical mechanisms that drive resistance.

Furthermore, we critically explore the challenges encountered in identifying reliable predictive biomarkers, understanding the evolutionary dynamics within the tumor microenvironment, and deciphering the mutation-driven resistance mechanisms and bypass signaling pathways that impede treatment efficacy. It is within these challenges that opportunities arise for the development of innovative therapeutic interventions and the formulation of novel treatment strategies.

Throughout this book, we underscore the paramount importance of multidisciplinary collaboration and the indispensable role of clinical trials. Collaboration serves as the catalyst for integrating diverse expertise and perspectives, fostering a comprehensive understanding of immunotherapy resistance, and propelling the development of effective solutions. Clinical trials, on the other hand, serve as the testing ground for novel approaches, enabling the validation of biomarkers, the evaluation of combination therapies, and the optimization of treatment regimens.

As we delve into the intricate mechanisms of resistance, we are constantly reminded of the patients and their families who navigate the arduous path of cancer treatment. Their unwavering courage, resilience, and hope serve as our driving force to unravel the complexities of resistance and develop innovative strategies that will ultimately enhance treatment outcomes and improve the lives of those affected by cancer.

This book is not merely a compendium of knowledge; it is a beacon of inspiration for medical professionals, researchers, and students engaged in the field of oncology. It aims to ignite scientific curiosity, stimulate further investigation, foster collaboration across disciplines, and drive the development of new therapeutic approaches. Our collective goal is to pave the way towards a future where the full potential of immunotherapy can be realized, offering renewed hope, brighter prospects, and improved quality of life for patients battling cancer.

May this book illuminate the intricacies of cancer immunotherapy resistance, serve as a compass for future research endeavors, and guide us toward a future where immunotherapy becomes a powerful weapon in the fight against cancer.

INTRODUCTION

Immunotherapy has revolutionized cancer treatment by harnessing the power of the immune system to fight against tumors. However, despite its remarkable success in some patients, resistance to immunotherapy remains a significant obstacle. Resistance mechanisms can hamper the effectiveness of immune-based treatments, leading to disease progression and limited therapeutic outcomes. Understanding the various factors and mechanisms underlying resistance to immunotherapy is crucial for developing strategies to overcome this challenge and improve patient outcomes.

I. Intrinsic Resistance
    A. Tumor cell-intrinsic factors
        1. Lack of tumor antigen expression
        2. Loss of antigen presentation machinery
        3. Alterations in antigen processing and presentation pathways
        4. Activation of pro-survival signaling pathways
    B. Tumor microenvironment factors

1. Immunosuppressive tumor microenvironment

2. Presence of inhibitory immune cells (e.g., regulatory T cells)

3. Secretion of immunosuppressive factors (e.g., TGF-β, IL-10)

4. Upregulation of immune checkpoint molecules

II. Acquired Resistance
  A. Tumor cell adaptations
    1. Neoantigen loss or downregulation
    2. Antigenic escape through immune editing
    3. Activation of alternative survival pathways
  B. Immune system exhaustion
    1. T cell dysfunction and exhaustion
    2. Upregulation of additional immune checkpoint molecules
    3. Inhibition of T cell trafficking to tumor sites
  C. Tumor heterogeneity and clonal evolution
    1. Emergence of resistant tumor cell clones
    2. Selection of immune-resistant phenotypes
    3. Evolutionary dynamics within the tumor microenvironment

III. Mechanisms of Resistance
  A. Genetic alterations
    1. Mutation-driven resistance mechanisms
    2. Activation of bypass signaling pathways
    3. Loss of antigen presentation machinery genes
  B. Epigenetic modifications

1. DNA methylation and histone modifications

2. Alterations in gene expression patterns

C. Immune evasion strategies

1. Upregulation of immune checkpoint molecules

2. Recruitment of suppressive immune cells

3. Modulation of the tumor microenvironment

IV. Overcoming Resistance to Immunotherapy

A. Combination therapies

1. Dual immune checkpoint blockade

2. Immune checkpoint inhibitors with targeted therapies

3. Combination of immunotherapy with other treatment modalities (chemotherapy, radiation)

B. Personalized medicine approaches

1. Identifying predictive biomarkers of response

2. Tailoring treatment strategies based on individual patient characteristics

C. Development of novel immunotherapeutic agents

1. Targeting alternative immune checkpoint pathways

2. Enhancing T cell function and activation

3. Improving antigen presentation and recognition

V. Future Directions and Conclusion

A. Advances in precision medicine and

genomics

    B. Novel therapeutic targets and approaches

    C.   Importance   of   multidisciplinary collaboration and clinical trials

    D. Concluding remarks on the ongoing efforts to overcome resistance to immunotherapy and improve cancer treatment outcomes

In conclusion, resistance to immunotherapy poses a significant challenge in the field of cancer treatment. Intrinsic and acquired resistance mechanisms can diminish the effectiveness of immune-based therapies. However, by unraveling the underlying mechanisms and developing innovative strategies, such as combination therapies and personalized medicine approaches, we can enhance the success of immunotherapy and pave the way for improved strategies for overcoming the associated challenges.

LACK OF TUMOR ANTIGEN EXPRESSION

Lack of tumor antigen expressionis a significant factor contributing to resistance to immunotherapy. Tumor antigens are proteins or other molecules expressed on the surface of cancer cells that can be recognized by the immune system as foreign, triggering an immune response. When tumor cells have limited or no expression of such antigens, they become less susceptible to immune recognition and destruction. Here are detailed notes on how the lack of tumor antigen expression can lead to resistance to immunotherapy:

1. Tumor Antigens:

  - Tumor antigens can be classified into two main types: tumor-specific antigens (TSAs) and tumor-associated antigens (TAAs).

  - TSAs are unique to tumor cells and are not expressed in normal cells, making them attractive targets for immune recognition and destruction.

  - TAAs, on the other hand, are also expressed in normal cells but are overexpressed or aberrantly expressed in tumor cells, making them potential targets for the immune system.

2. Loss or Downregulation of Tumor Antigens:

- Tumor cells can undergo genetic or epigenetic alterations that result in the loss or downregulation of tumor antigens.

- Genetic alterations, such as mutations or deletions in the genes encoding the antigens, can lead to the loss of antigen expression.

- Epigenetic modifications, such as DNA methylation or histone modifications, can silence the genes encoding the antigens, resulting in their downregulation or complete loss of expression.

3. Immune Escape Mechanisms:

- Lack of tumor antigen expression allows cancer cells to evade immune recognition and destruction.

- Without the presence of recognizable antigens, the immune system fails to mount an effective response against the tumor cells.

- Cancer cells can employ various immune escape mechanisms to avoid detection, such as altering antigen processing and presentation pathways or inhibiting the expression of major histocompatibility complex (MHC) molecules that present antigens to T cells.

4. Impact on Immunotherapeutic Strategies:

- Immunotherapeutic approaches, such as immune checkpoint inhibitors or adoptive cell therapies, rely on the recognition of tumor antigens by the immune system.

- In the absence of tumor antigens, these therapies may be ineffective as there are no targets for the immune response.

- Lack of tumor antigen expression limits the ability of immunotherapies to activate immune cells and initiate a robust anti-tumor immune response.

5. Overcoming Lack of Tumor Antigen Expression:

- Enhancing tumor antigen expression or presentation is a potential strategy to overcome resistance due to lack of antigen expression.

- Approaches such as epigenetic modulators or gene therapy techniques can be explored to restore or increase antigen expression on tumor cells.

- Identifying alternative tumor antigens that are expressed by a broader range of cancer cells or specific subsets of tumors can also expand the scope of immunotherapeutic targets.

In summary, the lack of tumor antigen expression is a significant hurdle in cancer immunotherapy. It prevents immune recognition and limits the effectiveness of immunotherapeutic approaches. Overcoming this resistance mechanism requires innovative strategies to restore or enhance tumor antigen expression, as well as the identification of alternative targets for immune recognition and destruction.

DR. BHRATRI BHUSHAN

LOSS OF ANTIGEN PRESENTATION MACHINERY

Loss of antigen presentation machinery is a crucial factor that can lead to resistance to cancer immunotherapy. The antigen presentation machinery plays a key role in presenting tumor antigens to immune cells, enabling them to recognize and mount an immune response against cancer cells. When the components of the antigen presentation machinery are impaired or absent, tumor cells become less susceptible to immune recognition and elimination. Here are detailed notes on how the loss of antigen presentation machinery can contribute to resistance to immunotherapy:

1. Antigen Presentation Machinery:
   - The antigen presentation machinery consists of various components involved in processing and presenting antigens to immune cells, primarily CD8+ cytotoxic T cells.
   - Major Histocompatibility Complex class I (MHC-I) molecules are a critical component of antigen presentation. They bind to processed

antigens and present them on the surface of cells for recognition by T cells.

- Antigen-processing machinery (APM) components, such as the proteasome, transporter associated with antigen processing (TAP), and the endoplasmic reticulum aminopeptidase (ERAP), are responsible for generating peptide fragments for MHC-I presentation.

2. Genetic Alterations and Loss of Antigen Presentation Machinery:

- Genetic alterations in genes encoding components of the antigen presentation machinery can lead to their loss or dysfunction.

- Mutations, deletions, or epigenetic modifications can disrupt the expression or function of MHC-I molecules and APM components.

- Heterozygous loss of MHC-I alleles or loss of heterozygosity (LOH) can result in reduced MHC-I expression on tumor cells.

- Alterations in APM components can impair antigen processing and peptide presentation, affecting the generation and presentation of tumor antigens.

3. Implications for Immunotherapy Resistance:

- Loss of antigen presentation machinery hampers the ability of tumor cells to present tumor antigens to immune cells.

- Without proper MHC-I expression and antigen processing, tumor cells escape immune recognition and destruction.

- Reduced MHC-I expression or impaired antigen processing leads to a weakened or ineffective anti-tumor immune response.

- Tumor cells lacking antigen presentation machinery may evade immune surveillance and remain undetected by immune cells.

4. Impact on Immunotherapeutic Strategies:

- Immunotherapeutic approaches, such as immune checkpoint inhibitors or adoptive cell therapies, rely on the recognition of tumor antigens presented through MHC-I molecules.

- Loss of antigen presentation machinery can render immunotherapies less effective or ineffective.

- Without proper antigen presentation, immune checkpoint inhibitors may fail to unleash the immune response, and adoptive cell therapies may encounter obstacles in antigen recognition and targeting.

5. Overcoming Loss of Antigen Presentation Machinery:

- Strategies to overcome the loss of antigen presentation machinery include enhancing MHC-I expression and restoring antigen processing.

- Approaches such as genetic engineering, epigenetic modulation, or targeted therapies can be explored to restore MHC-I expression on tumor cells.

- Augmenting antigen processing machinery

components or introducing exogenous components can help improve antigen processing and presentation.

In summary, the loss of antigen presentation machinery poses a significant challenge in cancer immunotherapy. It compromises the ability of tumor cells to present tumor antigens to the immune system, leading to immune evasion and resistance to immunotherapeutic approaches. Overcoming this resistance mechanism requires innovative strategies to restore or enhance antigen presentation machinery components, allowing effective immune recognition and activation against cancer cells.

ANTIGEN PROCESSING AND PRESENTATION PATHWAYS

Antigen processing and presentation pathways play a crucial role in cancer immunotherapy. These pathways are responsible for the generation of antigenic peptides from tumor antigens and their subsequent presentation on the surface of antigen-presenting cells (APCs) via Major Histocompatibility Complex (MHC) molecules. However, dysregulation or impairment of these pathways can contribute to resistance to immunotherapy. Here is a detailed discussion on antigen processing and presentation pathways and their implications for cancer immunotherapy resistance:

1. Antigen Processing Pathways:
   a. Proteasomal Degradation:
      - Tumor antigens are initially degraded into short peptide fragments by the proteasome.
      - The proteasome is a multi-subunit protease complex that selectively cleaves proteins into peptides.

- Dysfunctional or altered proteasomal activity can impact the generation of antigenic peptides.

b. Transporter Associated with Antigen Processing (TAP):
- After proteasomal degradation, peptide fragments are transported from the cytosol into the endoplasmic reticulum (ER) by TAP.
- TAP is responsible for the translocation of peptides into the ER, where they associate with MHC-I molecules.

c. Endoplasmic Reticulum Aminopeptidase (ERAP):
- ERAP trims the peptide fragments to optimal lengths for binding to MHC-I molecules.
- It ensures the generation of high-affinity peptides and contributes to MHC-I peptide repertoire diversity.
- Dysregulated ERAP activity can lead to alterations in peptide trimming, affecting antigen presentation.

2. Antigen Presentation Pathways:
a. MHC Class I Pathway:
- In the MHC class I pathway, peptides derived from intracellular proteins are presented on the cell surface by MHC class I molecules.
- MHC class I molecules consist of a peptide-binding groove and are expressed on the surface of most nucleated cells.

- Proper folding and assembly of MHC class I molecules with antigenic peptides are essential for efficient antigen presentation.

- Genetic alterations or abnormalities in MHC class I molecules can affect antigen presentation and immune recognition.

b. MHC Class II Pathway:

- The MHC class II pathway presents peptides derived from extracellular proteins on APCs, such as dendritic cells, macrophages, and B cells.

- Extracellular antigens are internalized via endocytosis or phagocytosis, processed in endosomes or lysosomes, and loaded onto MHC class II molecules.

- Dysregulation of MHC class II expression or impaired antigen processing in APCs can impact proper antigen presentation.

3. Implications for Immunotherapy Resistance:

a. Reduced Antigen Presentation:

- Dysfunctional antigen processing pathways can lead to reduced generation of antigenic peptides and subsequent MHC loading.

- Limited availability of tumor antigenic peptides hampers immune recognition and response against cancer cells.

b. Altered Peptide Repertoire:

- Dysregulated peptide trimming by ERAP or alterations in proteasomal degradation can affect the quality and diversity of presented peptides.

- Altered peptide repertoire can impact T cell receptor recognition and compromise immune responses.

c. Immune Escape Mechanisms:

- Dysfunctional antigen processing and presentation pathways can enable cancer cells to evade immune surveillance.
- Reduced or altered antigen presentation may prevent efficient activation of T cells and immune-mediated tumor elimination.

4. Overcoming Antigen Processing and Presentation Deficiencies:

a. Targeted Therapy:

- Therapeutic interventions targeting specific components of antigen processing pathways can restore their functionality.
- Strategies could include enhancing proteasomal activity, modulating ERAP function, or promoting efficient peptide transport via TAP.

b. Combinatorial Approaches:

- Combining immunotherapies with interventions that enhance antigen processing and presentation may improve treatment efficacy.
- For example, combining immune checkpoint inhibitors with agents that restore antigen presentation could synergistically enhance anti-tumor immune responses.

c. Personalized Vaccines:

- Development of personalized vaccines targeting patient-specific tumor antigens can bypass deficiencies in antigen processing and presentation pathways.

- Such vaccines can deliver antigenic peptides directly to APCs, ensuring effective antigen presentation and immune activation.

In conclusion, dysregulation or impairment of antigen processing and presentation pathways can contribute to resistance to cancer immunotherapy. Deficiencies in these pathways limit effective antigen presentation, impair T cell activation, and enable immune escape mechanisms. Overcoming these challenges requires targeted interventions, combinatorial approaches, and personalized vaccine strategies to restore or bypass deficiencies, enhancing the anti-tumor immune response and improving the outcomes of immunotherapeutic interventions.

ACTIVATION OF PRO-SURVIVAL AND SIGNALING PATHWAYS

Activation of pro-survival and signaling pathways is a significant contributor to resistance to cancer immunotherapy. Cancer cells can exploit various mechanisms to activate signaling pathways that promote their survival, growth, and immune evasion. These pathways often intersect with immune signaling, leading to resistance against immunotherapeutic interventions. Here are detailed notes on how the activation of pro-survival and signaling pathways can contribute to resistance to immunotherapy:

1. Activation of Pro-Survival Pathways:
   a. PI3K/Akt/mTOR Pathway:
   - The PI3K/Akt/mTOR pathway is frequently dysregulated in cancer and promotes cell survival, proliferation, and resistance to cell death.
   - Activation of this pathway can confer resistance to immunotherapy by inhibiting apoptosis, enhancing tumor cell survival, and dampening immune responses.

   b. MAPK/ERK Pathway:

- The MAPK/ERK pathway regulates cellular processes, including proliferation, survival, and differentiation.

- Activation of this pathway in cancer cells can promote tumor growth, survival, and resistance to immunotherapy.

c. NF-κB Pathway:

- The NF-κB pathway regulates immune responses, inflammation, and cell survival.

- Activation of NF-κB in cancer cells can confer resistance to apoptosis, promote immune evasion, and drive tumor progression.

2. Immune Signaling Crosstalk:

a. Immune Checkpoint Signaling:

- Immune checkpoint molecules, such as PD-1, PD-L1, CTLA-4, play a critical role in regulating immune responses and preventing excessive immune activation.

- Tumor cells can upregulate immune checkpoint molecules, creating an immunosuppressive microenvironment and inhibiting T cell-mediated anti-tumor responses.

b. JAK/STAT Pathway:

- The JAK/STAT pathway is involved in cytokine signaling and immune responses.

- Activation of this pathway in tumor cells can promote immune escape, suppress anti-tumor immune responses, and contribute to immunotherapy resistance.

c. TGF-β Signaling:
- TGF-β signaling pathway plays a complex role in cancer immunity, with both pro-tumorigenic and anti-tumorigenic effects.
- Aberrant activation of TGF-β signaling can promote immune suppression, induce regulatory T cells, and hinder anti-tumor immune responses.

3. Implications for Immunotherapy Resistance:
a. Enhanced Cell Survival and Resistance to Apoptosis:
- Activation of pro-survival pathways can protect cancer cells from immune-mediated cell death induced by immunotherapeutic approaches.
- Enhanced survival allows tumor cells to withstand immune attack, leading to treatment resistance.

b. Immune Evasion and Suppression:
- Activation of signaling pathways can contribute to an immunosuppressive tumor microenvironment, inhibiting immune cell function and antigen presentation.
- Immune evasion mechanisms, such as upregulation of immune checkpoint molecules or secretion of immunosuppressive factors, can compromise immunotherapy efficacy.

c. Resistance to T Cell-Mediated Cytotoxicity:
- Activation of pro-survival pathways in cancer cells can interfere with T cell cytotoxicity, impairing their ability to recognize and kill tumor

cells.

- Resistance to T cell-mediated cytotoxicity reduces the effectiveness of immunotherapeutic strategies that rely on T cell activation and tumor cell killing.

4. Overcoming Pro-Survival and Signaling Pathway Activation:

a. Combination Therapies:

- Combinations of immunotherapies with targeted therapies or inhibitors of pro-survival signaling pathways can overcome resistance mechanisms.

- Simultaneously targeting cancer cell survival pathways and enhancing immune responses can enhance treatment efficacy.

b. Targeted Inhibitors:

- Selective inhibitors of specific pro-survival or signaling pathways can be employed to block cancer cell survival signals and sensitize tumors to immunotherapy.

c. Biomarker-guided Approaches:

- Identification of predictive biomarkers associated with activation of pro-survival pathways can help stratify patients and personalize treatment strategies.

- Biomarker-guided approaches can improve patient selection and increase the likelihood of successful immunotherapy response.

In summary, the activation of pro-survival and

signaling pathways in cancer cells contributes to resistance against immunotherapy. Enhanced cell survival, immune evasion, and suppression, as well as interference with T cell cytotoxicity, are key consequences of pathway activation. Overcoming these resistance mechanisms requires a multi-faceted approach, including combination therapies, targeted inhibitors, and the use of biomarkers to guide treatment strategies. By disrupting pro-survival signaling and restoring immune responsiveness, the efficacy of immunotherapy can be improved, leading to better outcomes for cancer patients.

IMMUNOSUPPRESSIVE TUMOR MICROENVIRONMENT

The immunosuppressive tumor microenvironment (TME) is a critical factor contributing to resistance against cancer immunotherapy. The TME is a complex ecosystem composed of cancer cells, immune cells, stromal cells, and extracellular matrix components. Various immunosuppressive mechanisms within the TME can inhibit the anti-tumor immune response and limit the effectiveness of immunotherapeutic interventions. Here is a detailed discussion on how the immunosuppressive TME leads to resistance to immunotherapy:

1. Immune Cell Dysfunction:
   a. Regulatory T Cells (Tregs):
   - Tregs suppress immune responses and maintain immune tolerance.
   - Increased infiltration and activation of Tregs within the TME can suppress anti-tumor immune responses and hinder the effectiveness of immunotherapy.

b. Myeloid-Derived Suppressor Cells (MDSCs):

- MDSCs are a heterogeneous population of immune cells with immunosuppressive properties.

- MDSCs can inhibit T cell function, promote T cell exhaustion, and dampen anti-tumor immune responses within the TME.

c. Tumor-Associated Macrophages (TAMs):

- TAMs are polarized toward a pro-tumor M2 phenotype and exert immunosuppressive effects.

- M2 TAMs can inhibit T cell activation, promote angiogenesis, and contribute to an immunosuppressive TME.

d. Exhausted T Cells:

- Prolonged exposure to antigen stimulation within the TME can lead to T cell exhaustion, characterized by functional impairment and reduced effector functions.

- Exhausted T cells exhibit reduced cytokine production, decreased cytotoxicity, and increased expression of inhibitory receptors, limiting their ability to eliminate tumor cells.

2. Immune Checkpoint Pathways:

a. Programmed Cell Death Protein 1 (PD-1)/ Programmed Death Ligand 1 (PD-L1) Pathway:

- The interaction between PD-1 on T cells and PD-L1 on tumor cells or immune cells in the TME inhibits T cell activation and promotes immune tolerance.

- Upregulation of PD-L1 within the TME can prevent T cell-mediated tumor cell killing and contribute to immunotherapy resistance.

b. Cytotoxic T Lymphocyte-Associated Protein 4 (CTLA-4) Pathway:
- CTLA-4 is an inhibitory receptor expressed on T cells that competes with CD28 for binding to co-stimulatory molecules on antigen-presenting cells (APCs).
- CTLA-4 engagement attenuates T cell activation, reduces effector functions, and promotes immune suppression within the TME.

3. Immunosuppressive Factors:
a. Cytokines and Chemokines:
- The TME can produce various immunosuppressive cytokines and chemokines, such as transforming growth factor-beta (TGF-β) and interleukin-10 (IL-10).
- These factors can inhibit immune cell activation, induce T cell anergy, and promote immune tolerance.

b. Metabolic Reprogramming:
- Metabolic alterations within the TME, such as increased glycolysis and lactate production, can create an immunosuppressive environment.
- Metabolic byproducts and nutrient deprivation can impair T cell function and limit anti-tumor immune responses.

4. Implications for Immunotherapy Resistance:

a. Limited T Cell Infiltration and Function:

- The immunosuppressive TME restricts the infiltration and activation of effector T cells, reducing their ability to recognize and eliminate tumor cells.

- Impaired T cell function within the TME hampers the response to immunotherapeutic interventions.

b. Resistance to Immune Checkpoint Blockade:

- Upregulation of immune checkpoint molecules, such as PD-L1 and CTLA-4, within the TME can counteract the effects of immune checkpoint blockade therapies.

- Enhanced immunosuppressive signaling through checkpoint pathways can dampen T cell activation and attenuate the response to immunotherapy.

c. Lack of Antigen Presentation:

- The immunosuppressive TME can hamper antigen presentation by downregulating MHC molecules on tumor cells or impairing antigen processing and presentation pathways.

- Insufficient antigen presentation limits T cell recognition and reduces the effectiveness of immunotherapy.

5. Strategies to Overcome the Immunosuppressive TME:

a. Combination Therapies:

- Combining immunotherapies with agents that target immunosuppressive factors or pathways within the TME can overcome resistance.

- For example, combining immune checkpoint inhibitors with inhibitors of MDSCs or TAMs can enhance anti-tumor immune responses.

b. Modulation of TME Components:

- Targeting specific components of the TME, such as Tregs or TAMs, can alleviate immunosuppression and enhance the efficacy of immunotherapy.

c. Immunomodulatory Agents:

- The use of immunomodulatory agents, such as cytokines, immune stimulants, or inhibitors of immunosuppressive factors, can reverse immune suppression and promote anti-tumor responses.

In summary, the immunosuppressive TME creates a hostile environment for anti-tumor immune responses, leading to resistance against cancer immunotherapy. Dysfunctional immune cells, immune checkpoint pathways, immunosuppressive factors, and limited antigen presentation collectively contribute to immunotherapy resistance. Strategies targeting the immunosuppressive TME, including combination therapies and immunomodulatory agents, are being explored to overcome resistance and improve the effectiveness of immunotherapeutic interventions.

INHIBITORY IMMUNE CELLS

The presence of inhibitory immune cells,, particularly regulatory T cells (Tregs), plays a significant role in cancer immunotherapy resistance. Tregs are a specialized subset of immune cells that regulate immune responses and maintain immune tolerance. Within the tumor microenvironment (TME), Tregs can exert immunosuppressive effects, impair anti-tumor immune responses, and hinder the effectiveness of immunotherapeutic interventions. Here is a detailed discussion on how the presence of Tregs leads to cancer immunotherapy resistance:

1. Immunoregulatory Function of Tregs:
   a. Suppression of Effector T Cells:
      - Tregs can directly suppress the activation and effector functions of other immune cells, including CD4+ and CD8+ T cells, natural killer (NK) cells, and antigen-presenting cells (APCs).
      - Tregs achieve immunosuppression through the secretion of inhibitory cytokines (e.g., interleukin-10, TGF-β), direct cell-to-cell contact,

and metabolic disruption of effector cells.

b. Disruption of Tumor-Specific Immune Responses:
- Tregs can dampen tumor-specific immune responses by inhibiting the proliferation and activation of tumor-specific T cells.
- Tregs can also limit the production of pro-inflammatory cytokines and impair the cytotoxic functions of tumor-infiltrating lymphocytes.

2. Impact of Tregs on Immunotherapy Resistance:
a. Inhibition of Effector T Cell Responses:
- Tregs can suppress the activation and proliferation of effector T cells, limiting their ability to recognize and eliminate tumor cells.
- This suppression impairs the efficacy of immunotherapeutic interventions that rely on the activation and expansion of tumor-specific T cells.

b. Promotion of Tumor Immune Escape:
- Tregs facilitate immune evasion mechanisms employed by tumor cells.
- Tregs can upregulate immune checkpoint molecules (e.g., PD-1, CTLA-4) on effector T cells, resulting in their exhaustion and functional impairment.

c. Impaired Anti-Tumor Immune Surveillance:
- Tregs can hinder the immune system's ability to survey and control tumor growth.
- Their immunosuppressive activity within the TME allows tumor cells to evade immune

recognition and destruction.

3. Strategies to Counteract Treg-Mediated Immunotherapy Resistance:

a. Depletion or Functional Inhibition of Tregs:

- Targeting Tregs through selective depletion or functional inhibition can alleviate their immunosuppressive effects.

- This approach enhances the anti-tumor immune response and improves the efficacy of immunotherapy.

b. Treg Modulation:

- Modulating the activity or balance of Tregs within the TME can be explored to enhance anti-tumor immune responses.

- Strategies such as blocking Treg trafficking or altering their differentiation and activation may help overcome immunotherapy resistance.

c. Combination Therapies:

- Combining immunotherapies with agents that target Tregs, such as immune checkpoint inhibitors or Treg-specific antibodies, can synergistically enhance treatment outcomes.

- Simultaneously blocking immune checkpoint pathways and suppressing Treg-mediated immunosuppression can improve the anti-tumor immune response.

4. Biomarkers and Patient Selection:

- Identifying predictive biomarkers associated with Treg infiltration and activity can help guide patient selection and personalize treatment strategies.

- Biomarkers can aid in identifying patients who are more likely to benefit from Treg-targeted therapies or require combinatorial approaches.

In conclusion, the presence of inhibitory immune cells, particularly Tregs, within the TME contributes to cancer immunotherapy resistance. Tregs exert their immunosuppressive effects by suppressing effector T cell responses, promoting tumor immune escape, and impairing anti-tumor immune surveillance. Strategies aimed at depleting or modulating Tregs, as well as combination therapies, can help overcome Treg-mediated immunotherapy resistance and improve treatment outcomes for cancer patients. Additionally, the identification of relevant biomarkers can assist in patient selection and guide the use of Treg-targeted therapies in clinical practice.

SECRETION OF IMMUNOSUPPRESSIVE FACTORS

The secretion of immunosuppressive factors within the tumor microenvironment (TME) plays a crucial role in cancer immunotherapy resistance. Various cell types, including cancer cells, immune cells, and stromal cells, can secrete immunosuppressive factors that create an immunosuppressive milieu, impairing anti-tumor immune responses and limiting the effectiveness of immunotherapeutic interventions. Here is a detailed discussion on how the secretion of immunosuppressive factors leads to cancer immunotherapy resistance:

1. Cytokines and Chemokines:
    a. Transforming Growth Factor-beta (TGF-β):
        - TGF-β is a potent immunosuppressive cytokine that inhibits the proliferation and activation of immune cells.
        - TGF-β can promote the differentiation of regulatory T cells (Tregs) and myeloid-derived suppressor cells (MDSCs), which exert

immunosuppressive effects within the TME.

b. Interleukin-10 (IL-10):

- IL-10 is an immunosuppressive cytokine that inhibits the function of various immune cells, including T cells, NK cells, and APCs.

- Increased production of IL-10 within the TME can dampen anti-tumor immune responses and hinder the effectiveness of immunotherapy.

c. Indoleamine 2,3-dioxygenase (IDO):

- IDO is an enzyme that metabolizes tryptophan, leading to the depletion of this essential amino acid.

- IDO-mediated tryptophan depletion creates an immunosuppressive environment, inhibiting effector T cell function and promoting the expansion of Tregs.

2. Checkpoint Molecules:

a. Programmed Cell Death Ligand 1 (PD-L1):

- PD-L1 is expressed on tumor cells and certain immune cells within the TME.

- Interaction between PD-L1 and programmed cell death protein 1 (PD-1) on T cells inhibits T cell activation and promotes immune tolerance.

b. Cytotoxic T Lymphocyte-Associated Protein 4 (CTLA-4):

- CTLA-4 is an inhibitory receptor expressed on T cells that competes with CD28 for binding to co-stimulatory molecules on APCs.

- CTLA-4 engagement attenuates T cell

activation and dampens anti-tumor immune responses.

3. Metabolic Reprogramming:
  a. Lactate:
    - Cancer cells often exhibit enhanced glycolytic metabolism, leading to increased lactate production within the TME.
    - Accumulation of lactate creates an acidic and immunosuppressive microenvironment, impairing immune cell function.

  b. Adenosine:
    - Adenosine is generated in the TME through the degradation of adenosine triphosphate (ATP) released by dying cells.
    - Adenosine suppresses T cell activation and effector functions, promoting immune evasion by tumor cells.

4. Extracellular Matrix Components:
  a. Hyaluronic Acid (HA):
    - HA is an extracellular matrix component that can accumulate within the TME.
    - High levels of HA can create a physical barrier, impeding immune cell infiltration and limiting the efficacy of immunotherapeutic interventions.

5. Implications for Immunotherapy Resistance:
  a. Suppression of Anti-Tumor Immune Responses:
    - Immunosuppressive factors within the TME

can directly inhibit the activation, proliferation, and effector functions of immune cells, including T cells, NK cells, and APCs.

- Suppressed immune responses hamper the ability of the immune system to recognize and eliminate tumor cells, leading to immunotherapy resistance.

b. Induction of Immune Tolerance:

- Immunosuppressive factors promote the differentiation and expansion of Tregs and MDSCs, which suppress anti-tumor immune responses and promote immune tolerance.

- Enhanced immune tolerance within the TME limits the effectiveness of immunotherapeutic interventions.

6. Strategies to Overcome Immunotherapy Resistance Induced by Immunosuppressive Factors:

a. Immune Checkpoint Blockade:

- Blocking immune checkpoint pathways, such as PD-1/PD-L1 or CTLA-4, can alleviate the immunosuppressive effects mediated by checkpoint molecules.

b. Targeting Immunoregulatory Cells:

- Strategies aimed at depleting or modulating immunoregulatory cells, such as Tregs or MDSCs, can overcome their suppressive effects and enhance anti-tumor immune responses.

c. Combination Therapies:

- Combining immunotherapies with agents that target immunosuppressive factors or pathways can synergistically enhance treatment outcomes.

- Combination approaches can disrupt the immunosuppressive milieu and promote anti-tumor immune responses.

In conclusion, the secretion of immunosuppressive factors within the TME contributes to cancer immunotherapy resistance by inhibiting anti-tumor immune responses and promoting immune tolerance. Strategies aimed at targeting immunosuppressive factors, blocking immune checkpoint pathways, and modulating immunoregulatory cells can help overcome immunotherapy resistance induced by these factors. By disrupting the immunosuppressive environment, the efficacy of immunotherapeutic interventions can be improved, leading to better outcomes for cancer patients.

UPREGULATION OF IMMUNE CHECKPOINT MOLECULES

The upregulation of immune checkpoint molecules within the tumor microenvironment (TME) is a significant factor contributing to cancer immunotherapy resistance. Immune checkpoint molecules, such as programmed cell death protein 1 (PD-1), programmed death-ligand 1 (PD-L1), and cytotoxic T lymphocyte-associated protein 4 (CTLA-4), play a crucial role in regulating immune responses and maintaining immune tolerance. However, their overexpression or dysregulated activation within the TME can hinder anti-tumor immune responses and limit the effectiveness of immunotherapeutic interventions. Here is a detailed discussion on how the upregulation of immune checkpoint molecules leads to cancer immunotherapy resistance:

1. PD-1/PD-L1 Pathway:
   a. Tumor Expression of PD-L1:
      - Many tumor cells can upregulate PD-L1 expression in response to inflammatory signals

within the TME.

- Increased PD-L1 expression enables tumor cells to engage PD-1 on T cells, resulting in T cell exhaustion and functional impairment.

b. Induction of T Cell Exhaustion:

- Interaction between PD-1 on T cells and PD-L1 on tumor cells or other immune cells transmits inhibitory signals that suppress T cell activation and effector functions.

- T cell exhaustion reduces the ability of T cells to recognize and eliminate tumor cells, leading to immunotherapy resistance.

c. Adaptive Immune Resistance:

- Tumor cells can exploit the PD-1/PD-L1 pathway to evade immune surveillance and destruction.

- Upregulated PD-L1 expression allows tumor cells to evade recognition and destruction by T cells, promoting immune escape and treatment resistance.

2. CTLA-4 Pathway:

a. Inhibition of T Cell Activation:

- CTLA-4 competes with CD28 for binding to co-stimulatory molecules on antigen-presenting cells (APCs), resulting in the inhibition of T cell activation.

- CTLA-4 engagement dampens T cell responses, impairs the generation of effector T cells, and promotes immune tolerance.

b. Suppression of Anti-Tumor Immune Responses:

- Upregulation of CTLA-4 within the TME can suppress anti-tumor immune responses by inhibiting the priming and expansion of tumor-specific T cells.

- CTLA-4-mediated immunosuppression limits the efficacy of immunotherapeutic interventions that rely on T cell activation and expansion.

3. Implications for Immunotherapy Resistance:

a. Attenuation of T Cell Responses:

- The upregulation of immune checkpoint molecules negatively regulates T cell responses, leading to their attenuation and functional exhaustion.

- Attenuated T cell responses impair the ability to mount an effective anti-tumor immune response, contributing to immunotherapy resistance.

b. Promotion of Immune Tolerance:

- Increased expression of immune checkpoint molecules promotes immune tolerance within the TME.

- The engagement of immune checkpoint pathways inhibits the activation and function of immune cells, including T cells, NK cells, and APCs, resulting in a tolerogenic microenvironment.

4. Strategies to Overcome Immunotherapy

Resistance Induced by Immune Checkpoint Molecules:

a. Immune Checkpoint Blockade:

- Antibodies targeting immune checkpoint molecules, such as PD-1, PD-L1, and CTLA-4, can block inhibitory signaling and restore anti-tumor immune responses.

- Immune checkpoint blockade therapies aim to disrupt the interaction between checkpoint molecules and their ligands, enhancing the efficacy of immunotherapy.

b. Combination Therapies:

- Combining immune checkpoint inhibitors with other immunotherapeutic agents, such as vaccines, cytokines, or targeted therapies, can synergistically enhance treatment outcomes.

- Combination approaches can target multiple immunosuppressive mechanisms and promote a robust anti-tumor immune response.

c. Biomarkers and Patient Selection:

- Identifying predictive biomarkers, such as PD-L1 expression or tumor mutational burden, can help guide patient selection and personalize treatment strategies.

- Biomarkers can aid in identifying patients who are more likely to benefit from immune checkpoint blockade and optimize treatment outcomes.

In conclusion, the upregulation of immune

checkpoint molecules within the TME contributes to cancer immunotherapy resistance by attenuating T cell responses, promoting immune tolerance, and facilitating immune escape by tumor cells. Strategies targeting immune checkpoint molecules, such as immune checkpoint blockade and combination therapies, offer promising approaches to overcome immunotherapy resistance induced by the upregulation of these molecules. Understanding the complex interactions between immune checkpoints and the TME is crucial for developing effective immunotherapeutic interventions and improving outcomes for cancer patients.

NEOANTIGENS

Neoantigens,, which are tumor-specific antigens derived from somatic mutations, play a critical role in cancer immunotherapy by serving as targets for the immune system. However, the loss or downregulation of neoantigens within the tumor cells can contribute to cancer immunotherapy resistance. Here is a detailed discussion on how neoantigen loss or downregulation leads to resistance to cancer immunotherapy:

1. Immune Recognition of Neoantigens:
   a. Tumor-Specific T Cell Responses:
   - Neoantigens are recognized by T cells as foreign antigens, leading to the activation of tumor-specific T cell responses.
   - Tumor-infiltrating lymphocytes (TILs) or tumor-specific T cells can recognize and eliminate tumor cells expressing neoantigens.

   b. Immune Checkpoint Regulation:
   - Neoantigen recognition can trigger immune checkpoint pathways, such as PD-1/PD-L1, leading to the regulation of T cell responses.

- Immune checkpoint molecules can modulate the intensity and duration of T cell activation in response to neoantigens.

2. Mechanisms of Neoantigen Loss or Downregulation:

a. Immune Editing:

- The immune system exerts selective pressure on tumor cells, leading to the outgrowth of cells that have escaped immune recognition.

- Tumor cells with low or absent neoantigen expression have a survival advantage, as they evade immune attack.

b. Loss of Heterozygosity:

- Tumor cells can lose one copy of a gene carrying a neoantigen through loss of heterozygosity (LOH), resulting in reduced neoantigen presentation.

- LOH events can occur during tumor evolution and contribute to the loss or downregulation of neoantigens.

c. Epigenetic Silencing:

- Epigenetic modifications, such as DNA methylation or histone modifications, can lead to the silencing of genes encoding neoantigens.

- Epigenetic alterations can affect the expression or presentation of neoantigens, making tumor cells less visible to the immune system.

d. Alternative Splicing:

- Tumor cells can employ alternative splicing mechanisms to produce isoforms that lack neoantigens or have altered antigenic properties.

- Altered splicing events can result in the loss or modification of neoantigen presentation, reducing immune recognition.

3. Implications for Immunotherapy Resistance:

a. Reduced T Cell Recognition:

- Loss or downregulation of neoantigens diminishes T cell recognition and reduces the ability of the immune system to target tumor cells effectively.

- Tumor cells with low neoantigen expression evade immune surveillance and exhibit decreased susceptibility to immunotherapy.

b. Limitations of Targeted Therapies:

- Neoantigen loss or downregulation can undermine the effectiveness of targeted therapies that rely on specific neoantigen-targeted mechanisms.

- Reduced neoantigen presentation limits the therapeutic response to targeted agents designed to exploit neoantigen vulnerabilities.

4. Strategies to Overcome Neoantigen Loss or Downregulation:

a. Personalized Vaccines:

- Personalized cancer vaccines can be designed based on individual neoantigen profiles to induce neoantigen-specific immune responses.

- Vaccines can boost the immune recognition of existing neoantigens or elicit responses against newly emerging neoantigens.

b. Combination Therapies:

- Combining immunotherapies, such as immune checkpoint inhibitors or adoptive cell therapies, with other treatment modalities can enhance the anti-tumor immune response.
- Combination approaches may help overcome neoantigen loss by targeting alternative immune evasion mechanisms or enhancing overall immune activation.

c. Monitoring and Adaptation:

- Regular monitoring of tumor neoantigen profiles can provide insights into changes in antigen expression over time.
- Adjusting treatment strategies based on evolving neoantigen landscapes can help overcome resistance and improve treatment outcomes.

In conclusion, the loss or downregulation of neoantigens within tumor cells represents a mechanism of resistance to cancer immunotherapy. Strategies aimed at personalized vaccines, combination therapies, and adaptive treatment approaches can help overcome neoantigen loss or downregulation by enhancing immune recognition and targeting alternative immune evasion mechanisms. Understanding the dynamic nature of neoantigen expression and implementing tailored therapeutic approaches are crucial for maximizing the efficacy of immunotherapy in the face of neoantigen loss.

ANTIGEN ESCAPE

Antigen escape through immune editing is a phenomenon in which tumor cells undergo genetic alterations or selection processes to evade immune recognition and elimination. This process can contribute to resistance to cancer immunotherapy. Here is a detailed discussion on how antigen escape through immune editing leads to resistance to cancer immunotherapy:

1. Immune Editing:
   a. Elimination Phase:
      - The immune system recognizes tumor cells expressing antigens, including neoantigens, and eliminates them through immune responses.
      - Tumor cells with high immunogenicity and antigen expression are targeted and destroyed by immune cells.

   b. Equilibrium Phase:
      - During this phase, tumor cells that are not eliminated enter a dynamic equilibrium with the immune system.
      - Immune responses control tumor growth,

but some tumor cells with reduced antigen expression or immune evasion mechanisms survive.

c. Escape Phase:

- Tumor cells that have acquired genetic alterations or immune evasion mechanisms gain a selective advantage and escape immune recognition.

- These escaped tumor cells are resistant to immune-mediated elimination and contribute to tumor progression.

2. Mechanisms of Antigen Escape through Immune Editing:

a. Downregulation of Antigen Expression:

- Tumor cells can downregulate the expression of antigens, including neoantigens, to avoid recognition by immune cells.

- Genetic alterations or epigenetic modifications can lead to reduced antigen expression, rendering tumor cells invisible to the immune system.

b. Loss of Antigen Presentation Machinery:

- Alterations in the antigen presentation machinery, such as defects in the expression or function of major histocompatibility complex (MHC) molecules, can impair antigen presentation.

- Tumor cells with compromised antigen presentation machinery are less likely to be recognized by T cells, enabling their escape from immune surveillance.

   c. Immune Suppressive Factors:
   - Immunosuppressive factors secreted by tumor cells or immune cells in the tumor microenvironment can inhibit immune responses and facilitate antigen escape.
   - Factors such as cytokines, chemokines, and regulatory immune cells create an immunosuppressive milieu that hampers anti-tumor immune activity.

3. Implications for Immunotherapy Resistance:
   a. Loss of Targetable Antigens:
   - Antigen escape through immune editing reduces the availability of targetable antigens for immunotherapies, limiting their efficacy.
   - Tumor cells with decreased antigen expression or alterations in antigen presentation machinery become resistant to antigen-specific immunotherapies.

   b. Immune Tolerance and Suppression:
   - Immune escape mechanisms contribute to the development of an immunosuppressive tumor microenvironment, leading to immune tolerance and suppression.
   - Suppressive factors and regulatory immune cells inhibit the effector functions of immune cells, compromising the effectiveness of immunotherapeutic interventions.

4. Strategies to Overcome Antigen Escape:

a. Combination Immunotherapies:

- Combining multiple immunotherapeutic approaches, such as immune checkpoint inhibitors, adoptive cell therapies, or targeted therapies, can target different aspects of immune escape.

- Combination therapies can enhance immune responses, overcome immune evasion mechanisms, and improve treatment outcomes.

b. Personalized Vaccines:

- Personalized cancer vaccines targeting a broad range of antigens, including neoantigens, can overcome antigen escape by stimulating a robust immune response.

- Vaccines can help broaden the immune repertoire and target diverse tumor antigens, reducing the likelihood of antigen escape.

c. Monitoring and Adaptive Treatment:

- Regular monitoring of tumor antigen profiles and immune responses can guide treatment decisions and adaptation strategies.

- Adjusting treatment approaches based on evolving antigen landscapes can help overcome antigen escape and improve therapeutic outcomes.

In conclusion, antigen escape through immune editing is a significant mechanism contributing to resistance to cancer immunotherapy. Tumor cells employ various strategies, such as downregulation of antigen expression, loss of antigen presentation machinery, and immune suppression, to evade immune recognition and elimination. Overcoming antigen escape requires the development of combinatorial approaches, personalized vaccines, and adaptive treatment strategies to target multiple escape mechanisms and restore effective anti-tumor immune responses. Understanding the dynamic interplay between tumor cells and the immune system is crucial for developing strategies to overcome antigen escape and improve the success of cancer immunotherapy.

ACTIVATION OF ALTERNATIVE SURVIVAL PATHWAYS

Activation of alternative survival pathways in cancer cells can confer resistance to immunotherapy. When confronted with immune-mediated attack, cancer cells can activate various survival mechanisms that promote cell survival, immune evasion, and resistance to therapeutic interventions. Here is a detailed discussion on how the activation of alternative survival pathways leads to resistance to cancer immunotherapy:

1. Activation of Anti-apoptotic Pathways:

    a. Upregulation of Bcl-2 Family Proteins:

       - Cancer cells may upregulate anti-apoptotic proteins, such as Bcl-2, Bcl-XL, and Mcl-1, to inhibit apoptosis triggered by immune-mediated cytotoxicity.

       - Increased expression of these proteins confers resistance to immune-induced cell death and promotes cancer cell survival.

    b. Activation of Survival Signaling Pathways:

       - Cancer cells can activate survival signaling

pathways, such as the PI3K/AKT and MAPK/ERK pathways, in response to immune attack.

- Activation of these pathways enhances cell survival, prevents apoptosis, and promotes resistance to immunotherapy.

2. Epithelial-Mesenchymal Transition (EMT):

  a. Acquisition of Mesenchymal Phenotype:

- Cancer cells undergoing EMT transition from an epithelial to a mesenchymal phenotype, promoting invasiveness and immune evasion.

- EMT-associated changes, such as downregulation of epithelial markers (e.g., E-cadherin) and upregulation of mesenchymal markers (e.g., N-cadherin, vimentin), contribute to immunotherapy resistance.

  b. Immune Evasion:

- EMT can confer resistance to immune-mediated cytotoxicity by downregulating components involved in antigen presentation and recognition.

- Reduced expression of major histocompatibility complex (MHC) molecules and immune checkpoint molecules on mesenchymal-like cancer cells hinders immune recognition and promotes resistance.

3. Activation of DNA Damage Response (DDR) Pathways:

  a. Enhanced DNA Repair:

- Cancer cells with activated DDR pathways

exhibit enhanced DNA repair mechanisms, enabling them to survive DNA damage induced by immune-mediated cytotoxicity.

- Efficient DNA repair reduces the efficacy of DNA-damaging agents, including immune-mediated cytotoxicity, contributing to therapy resistance.

b. Activation of Checkpoint Signaling:

- Activation of checkpoint signaling pathways, such as the ATM/ATR pathway and the p53 pathway, promotes cell cycle arrest, DNA repair, and cell survival.

- Checkpoint activation enables cancer cells to overcome DNA damage-induced cell death and evade immune attack.

4. Metabolic Adaptation:

a. Reprogramming of Energy Metabolism:

- Cancer cells may undergo metabolic reprogramming, such as increased aerobic glycolysis (the Warburg effect), to meet their energy demands and promote survival.

- Altered metabolism can provide a growth advantage to cancer cells and contribute to immune evasion and therapy resistance.

b. Nutrient Competition:

- Tumor cells can outcompete immune cells for essential nutrients, such as glucose and amino acids, within the tumor microenvironment.

- Nutrient competition creates

an immunosuppressive environment and compromises immune cell function, leading to immunotherapy resistance.

5. Implications for Immunotherapy Resistance:
  a. Reduced Cell Death:
   - Activation of alternative survival pathways in cancer cells limits immune-induced cell death, reducing the efficacy of immunotherapy.
   - Enhanced cell survival mechanisms counteract the cytotoxic effects of immune effector cells, leading to resistance.

  b. Persistent Tumor Growth and Progression:
   - Activation of alternative survival pathways promotes tumor cell survival and allows the continued growth and progression of resistant cancer cells.
   - Enhanced survival mechanisms

enable tumor cells to withstand immune-mediated attack, leading to treatment failure.

6. Strategies to Overcome Alternative Survival Pathways:
  a. Combination Therapies:
   - Combination approaches targeting both cancer cell survival pathways and immunotherapy can synergistically overcome resistance.
   - Simultaneously inhibiting alternative survival pathways while enhancing immune responses can improve treatment outcomes.

b. Targeted Therapies:

- Targeted inhibitors against specific survival pathways, such as PI3K/AKT, MAPK/ERK, or Bcl-2 family proteins, can sensitize cancer cells to immune-mediated cytotoxicity.

- Inhibiting alternative survival pathways can restore vulnerability to immunotherapy and enhance treatment efficacy.

c. Metabolic Modulation:

- Modulating cancer cell metabolism, such as targeting key metabolic enzymes or nutrient transporters, can disrupt metabolic adaptations and sensitize cancer cells to immunotherapy.

- Combining metabolic inhibitors with immunotherapeutic agents can overcome immunotherapy resistance mediated by metabolic reprogramming.

In conclusion, the activation of alternative survival pathways in cancer cells contributes to resistance to immunotherapy. Understanding these survival mechanisms and developing strategies to target them, either alone or in combination with immunotherapies, is crucial for overcoming resistance and improving treatment outcomes for cancer patients.

T CELL DYSFUNCTION
AND EXHAUSTION

T cell dysfunction and exhaustion are key factors contributing to resistance to cancer immunotherapy. T cells play a crucial role in recognizing and eliminating tumor cells, but their functionality can be compromised within the tumor microenvironment, leading to resistance. Here is a detailed discussion on how T cell dysfunction and exhaustion contribute to resistance to cancer immunotherapy:

1. T Cell Dysfunction:
   a. Impaired T Cell Activation:
   - Tumor cells and the immunosuppressive tumor microenvironment can inhibit the activation of T cells, impairing their ability to mount an effective immune response.
   - Reduced T cell activation limits their cytotoxic functions and cytokine production required for tumor cell elimination.

   b. Defective Antigen Recognition:
   - Tumor cells may downregulate or alter the expression of antigens, leading to ineffective

recognition by T cells.

- Defective antigen recognition hinders T cell-mediated targeting and killing of tumor cells, promoting resistance.

c. Altered Co-stimulation:

- Co-stimulatory signals necessary for full T cell activation, such as CD28-mediated signaling, can be inhibited or dysregulated within the tumor microenvironment.

- Insufficient co-stimulation results in suboptimal T cell activation, reducing their effector functions and impeding anti-tumor responses.

2. T Cell Exhaustion:

a. Continuous Antigen Stimulation:

- Prolonged exposure to persistent antigens, such as tumor-associated antigens, can lead to T cell exhaustion.

- Chronic antigen stimulation induces a progressive loss of effector functions and upregulation of inhibitory receptors on T cells.

b. Upregulation of Inhibitory Receptors:

- Exhausted T cells express inhibitory receptors, such as PD-1, CTLA-4, TIM-3, and LAG-3, which dampen their activation and effector functions.

- Increased inhibitory receptor expression limits T cell cytotoxicity and cytokine production, reducing their ability to control tumor growth.

c. Dysfunctional Signaling Pathways:
- Exhausted T cells exhibit dysregulated signaling pathways, including impaired TCR signaling and altered metabolic pathways.
- Dysfunctional signaling impairs T cell effector functions and proliferation, contributing to immunotherapy resistance.

3. Immunosuppressive Factors:
a. Immune Checkpoint Ligands:
- Tumor cells and immune cells within the tumor microenvironment express ligands, such as PD-L1 and CTLA-4, that engage inhibitory receptors on T cells.
- Engagement of these checkpoint ligands promotes T cell exhaustion and dampens anti-tumor responses.

b. Immunosuppressive Cytokines:
- The tumor microenvironment can produce immunosuppressive cytokines, such as TGF-β and IL-10, which inhibit T cell activation and promote exhaustion.
- Increased levels of immunosuppressive cytokines impair T cell function and contribute to resistance to immunotherapy.

4. Implications for Immunotherapy Resistance:
a. Reduced Tumor Cell Killing:
- Dysfunctional and exhausted T cells have impaired cytotoxicity, limiting their ability to eliminate tumor cells.

- T cell dysfunction and exhaustion reduce the efficacy of immunotherapy, as the immune system fails to effectively target and eliminate tumor cells.

b. Immune Evasion and Survival:

- T cell dysfunction and exhaustion enable tumor cells to evade immune surveillance and establish an immunosuppressive microenvironment.

- Immunosuppressive factors and inhibitory receptor signaling promote tumor cell survival and growth, contributing to immunotherapy resistance.

5. Strategies to Overcome T Cell Dysfunction and Exhaustion:

a. Immune Checkpoint Blockade:

- Blocking inhibitory receptors, such as PD-1, CTLA-4, or TIM-3, with checkpoint inhibitors can reinvigorate exhausted T cells and restore their anti-tumor functions.

- Immune checkpoint blockade can reverse T cell dysfunction and enhance immunotherapy efficacy.

b. Combination Therapies:

- Combining immune checkpoint inhibitors with other immunotherapeutic approaches, such as adoptive cell therapy or cancer vaccines, can enhance T cell function and overcome exhaustion.

- Combination therapies target multiple pathways and provide synergistic effects to overcome resistance.

c. Targeting Immunoregulatory Factors:

- Inhibiting immunosuppressive cytokines or immune checkpoint ligands within the tumor microenvironment can disrupt immunosuppression and restore T cell function.

- Modulating the immunosuppressive factors enhances the anti-tumor immune response and improves immunotherapy outcomes.

In conclusion, T cell dysfunction and exhaustion contribute to resistance to cancer immunotherapy by impairing T cell activation, reducing effector functions, and promoting immune evasion within the tumor microenvironment. Overcoming T cell dysfunction and exhaustion through immune checkpoint blockade, combination therapies, and targeting immunoregulatory factors is crucial for improving the effectiveness of immunotherapy and overcoming resistance.

UPREGULATION OF ADDITIONAL IMMUNE CHECKPOINT MOLECULES

Upregulation of additional immune checkpoint molecules can contribute to resistance to cancer immunotherapy. Immune checkpoint molecules play a crucial role in regulating immune responses and maintaining self-tolerance. However, tumor cells can exploit these checkpoints by upregulating additional inhibitory receptors, creating an immunosuppressive environment that hinders effective anti-tumor immune responses. Here is a detailed discussion on how the upregulation of additional immune checkpoint molecules leads to resistance to cancer immunotherapy:

1. Increased Expression of Inhibitory Receptors:
   a. PD-L1:
      - Programmed Death-Ligand 1 (PD-L1) is upregulated on tumor cells in response to inflammatory signals within the tumor microenvironment.
      - Increased expression of PD-L1 interacts with

PD-1 on T cells, inhibiting their effector functions and promoting immune evasion.

b. LAG-3 (Lymphocyte Activation Gene 3):

- LAG-3 is an inhibitory receptor expressed on T cells that negatively regulates T cell activation and function.

- Tumor cells can upregulate LAG-3, leading to T cell exhaustion and impaired anti-tumor responses.

c. TIGIT (T cell Immunoreceptor with Ig and ITIM Domains):

- TIGIT is an inhibitory receptor expressed on T cells that competes with the co-stimulatory receptor CD226 (DNAM-1) for binding to common ligands, such as CD155 (PVR) and CD112 (PVRL2).

- Upregulation of TIGIT on T cells suppresses their cytotoxicity and cytokine production, contributing to immunotherapy resistance.

d. TIM-3 (T cell Immunoglobulin and Mucin-domain containing-3):

- TIM-3 is an inhibitory receptor expressed on T cells that regulates immune responses.

- Increased TIM-3 expression on T cells is associated with T cell exhaustion and reduced anti-tumor immunity.

e. VISTA (V-domain Ig suppressor of T cell Activation):

- VISTA is an inhibitory receptor expressed on immune cells, including T cells and antigen-presenting cells.

- Upregulation of VISTA in the tumor microenvironment suppresses T cell activation and promotes immune tolerance.

2. Implications for Immunotherapy Resistance:

a. Enhanced Immune Suppression:

- Upregulation of additional immune checkpoint molecules further enhances immune suppression and inhibits anti-tumor immune responses.

- Increased expression of inhibitory receptors dampens T cell activation and function, leading to reduced tumor cell killing.

b. Combinatorial Effects:

- The simultaneous upregulation of multiple immune checkpoint molecules creates a network of inhibitory signals that reinforce immune suppression.

- Combinatorial effects make it more challenging for immunotherapies targeting a single immune checkpoint to achieve effective tumor control.

3. Strategies to Overcome Upregulated Immune Checkpoints:

a. Combination Immunotherapy:

- Combining multiple immune checkpoint inhibitors that target different checkpoint molecules can overcome resistance driven by upregulated immune checkpoints.

- Simultaneously blocking multiple inhibitory receptors enhances T cell activation and promotes anti-tumor immune responses.

b. Dual Blockade:
- Dual blockade refers to the simultaneous targeting of a checkpoint receptor and its corresponding ligand, such as PD-1/PD-L1 or LAG-3/PD-L1.
- Dual blockade can disrupt the inhibitory signaling between tumor cells and T cells, restoring T cell function and enhancing immunotherapy efficacy.

c. Novel Checkpoint Inhibitors:
- Developing novel checkpoint inhibitors that target upregulated immune checkpoints, such as LAG-3, TIGIT, TIM-3, and VISTA, holds promise for overcoming resistance.
- Novel inhibitors can reverse T cell exhaustion and enhance anti-tumor immune responses.

In summary, upregulation of additional immune checkpoint molecules by tumor cells contributes to resistance to cancer immunotherapy. The enhanced immune suppression and combinatorial effects of multiple inhibitory receptors hinder effective anti-tumor immune responses. Overcoming this resistance can be achieved through combination immunotherapy, dual blockade strategies, and the development of novel checkpoint inhibitors. By targeting multiple immune checkpoints simultaneously, we can restore T cell function and improve the outcomes of cancer immunotherapy.

INHIBITION OF T CELL
TRAFFICKING TO TUMOR SITES

Inhibition of T cell trafficking to tumor sites is a significant factor contributing to resistance against cancer immunotherapy. T cells play a crucial role in recognizing and eliminating tumor cells, but their ability to reach the tumor microenvironment is often impaired. Here is a detailed discussion on how inhibition of T cell trafficking leads to resistance to cancer immunotherapy:

1. Chemokine Signaling and Adhesion Molecules:
    a. Chemokines:
        - Chemokines are small signaling proteins that guide immune cell migration to specific tissues and organs.
        - Tumor cells can produce chemokines that divert T cells away from the tumor site or recruit immunosuppressive cells that hinder T cell function.

    b. Adhesion Molecules:
        - Adhesion molecules facilitate the interaction between immune cells and endothelial cells,

allowing their transmigration into tissues.

- Tumor cells can upregulate adhesion molecules that trap T cells in the peripheral circulation or prevent their infiltration into the tumor site.

2. Tumor Vasculature and Extracellular Matrix (ECM):

a. Abnormal Tumor Vasculature:

- Tumor blood vessels can have irregular structures and leakiness, impairing T cell extravasation and infiltration into the tumor.

- Poor perfusion and reduced oxygenation within the tumor microenvironment further hamper T cell migration and function.

b. Remodeled ECM:

- Tumor cells can modify the ECM composition and stiffness, creating physical barriers that limit T cell infiltration.

- Increased collagen deposition and matrix remodeling prevent T cells from reaching tumor cells, leading to resistance against immunotherapy.

3. Immunosuppressive Factors:

a. Immune Checkpoint Ligands:

- Tumor cells and immune cells within the tumor microenvironment can express immune checkpoint ligands, such as PD-L1, that inhibit T cell trafficking and infiltration.

- Engagement of immune checkpoint

receptors on T cells prevents their migration into the tumor site.

b. Immunosuppressive Cytokines:
- Immunoregulatory cytokines, such as TGF-β and IL-10, produced by tumor cells and immune cells in the tumor microenvironment, can impair T cell trafficking.
- These cytokines alter chemokine gradients, inhibit adhesion molecule expression, and hinder T cell migration to the tumor site.

4. Implications for Immunotherapy Resistance:
a. Reduced Tumor Infiltration:
- Inhibition of T cell trafficking limits their access to tumor cells, reducing their ability to recognize and eliminate malignant cells.
- Insufficient T cell infiltration into the tumor microenvironment impedes the efficacy of immunotherapeutic interventions.

b. Immune Privileged Tumor Niches:
- Tumors can establish immune privileged niches where immune cells, including T cells, have limited access.
- These niches shield tumor cells from immune surveillance and promote tumor immune evasion, leading to therapy resistance.

5. Strategies to Overcome T Cell Trafficking Inhibition:
a. Chemokine Modulation:
- Modulating the chemokine profile within

the tumor microenvironment can promote T cell recruitment and infiltration.

- Administering exogenous chemokines or modifying the expression of specific chemokines can enhance T cell trafficking to tumor sites.

b. Vascular Normalization:

- Agents targeting abnormal tumor vasculature can normalize blood vessels, improve perfusion, and enhance T cell infiltration.

- Promoting vascular normalization facilitates the delivery of T cells to the tumor and improves immunotherapy outcomes.

c. ECM Remodeling:

- Strategies aimed at remodeling the ECM, such as enzymatic degradation or inhibition of ECM-modifying enzymes, can facilitate T cell migration into the tumor.

- Disrupting physical barriers created by the ECM improves T cell infiltration and enhances the efficacy of immunotherapies.

d. Combination Therapies:

- Combining approaches that address T cell trafficking inhibition with immunotherapeutic interventions can overcome resistance.

- Combining checkpoint inhibitors with agents targeting T cell trafficking barriers synergistically enhances T cell infiltration and anti-tumor responses.

In conclusion, inhibition of T cell trafficking

to tumor sites represents a significant obstacle to successful cancer immunotherapy. Modulating chemokine signaling, targeting abnormal tumor vasculature and ECM, and addressing immunosuppressive factors can help overcome T cell trafficking inhibition. Implementing combination therapies that enhance T cell infiltration, along with immunotherapeutic interventions, is crucial for overcoming resistance and improving the effectiveness of cancer immunotherapy.

EMERGENCE OF RESISTANT TUMOR CELL CLONES

The emergence of resistant tumor cell clones is a major factor contributing to cancer immunotherapy resistance. Tumors are composed of heterogeneous cell populations, and within this complexity, certain tumor cell clones can acquire mechanisms to evade immune recognition and elimination. Here is a detailed discussion on how the emergence of resistant tumor cell clones leads to resistance against cancer immunotherapy:

1. Tumor Cell Heterogeneity:
   a. Clonal Evolution:
      - Tumors exhibit genetic and phenotypic heterogeneity, resulting from genetic mutations, genomic instability, and clonal selection.
      - Within this heterogeneity, some tumor cell clones may possess inherent or acquired resistance mechanisms against immune-mediated elimination.

   b. Selection Pressure:
      - Immunotherapy exerts selective pressure on

tumors by targeting specific antigens or immune checkpoints.

- Under this pressure, tumor cells with pre-existing or acquired resistance traits have a survival advantage and can outcompete susceptible tumor cells.

2. Mechanisms of Resistance:
   a. Antigen Loss or Downregulation:

- Resistant tumor cell clones may lose or downregulate the expression of antigens targeted by immune cells, making them invisible to the immune system.

- Lack of target antigens prevents efficient recognition and elimination of tumor cells by immune effectors.

   b. Alterations in Antigen Processing and Presentation:

- Resistant clones can acquire mutations that disrupt antigen processing and presentation pathways, hampering the generation of tumor-specific antigens.

- Impaired antigen presentation reduces the ability of immune cells to recognize and mount an immune response against tumor cells.

   c. Immune Checkpoint Upregulation:

- Resistant tumor cell clones may upregulate immune checkpoint molecules, such as PD-L1 or CTLA-4, to inhibit T cell activation and evade immune surveillance.

- Increased checkpoint expression provides a shield against immune attack and reduces the effectiveness of immunotherapy.

d. Altered Signaling Pathways:
- Resistant tumor cell clones can activate alternative signaling pathways that promote cell survival, growth, and immune evasion.
- Dysregulated signaling pathways contribute to tumor cell resistance and render immunotherapy less effective.

e. Immunomodulatory Factors:
- Resistant clones may secrete immunosuppressive factors, such as cytokines or chemokines, that create an immunosuppressive tumor microenvironment.
- The presence of immunomodulatory factors dampens immune responses, inhibits effector functions of immune cells, and promotes therapy resistance.

3. Implications for Immunotherapy Resistance:
a. Persistence of Resistant Clones:
- Resistant tumor cell clones have a survival advantage and can continue to proliferate and expand within the tumor.
- The persistence of resistant clones compromises the effectiveness of immunotherapy by allowing tumor growth and progression.

b. Treatment Failure and Disease Recurrence:
- The presence of resistant tumor cell

clones can lead to treatment failure and disease recurrence, as these cells evade immune elimination and drive disease progression.

- Resistant clones can repopulate the tumor and contribute to the development of metastases.

4. Strategies to Overcome Resistant Tumor Cell Clones:

a. Combination Therapies:

- Combining different immunotherapeutic approaches, such as immune checkpoint inhibitors, adoptive cell therapy, or targeted therapies, can target multiple resistance mechanisms simultaneously.

- Combination therapies increase the likelihood of eliminating resistant clones and improve overall treatment efficacy.

b. Personalized Medicine:

- Incorporating genomic profiling and molecular characterization of tumors enables the identification of specific resistance mechanisms in individual patients.

- Personalized treatment approaches can then be designed to target the identified resistance mechanisms and overcome therapy resistance.

c. Early Detection and Intervention:

- Monitoring tumor response and identifying emerging resistance during treatment allows for timely intervention.

- Early detection of resistant clones can guide

treatment modifications and the implementation of combination therapies to prevent disease progression.

In conclusion, the emergence of resistant tumor cell clones poses a significant challenge to cancer immunotherapy. Tumor cell heterogeneity, coupled with the selective pressure exerted by immunotherapy, leads to the survival and expansion of resistant clones. Understanding the underlying mechanisms of resistance and implementing strategies such as combination therapies and personalized medicine can help overcome resistance, improve treatment outcomes, and prevent disease recurrence.

SELECTION OF IMMUNE-RESISTANT PHENOTYPES

The selection of immune-resistant phenotypes is a crucial factor contributing to cancer immunotherapy resistance. As tumors evolve and interact with the immune system, certain phenotypes can emerge that evade immune recognition and elimination. Here is a detailed discussion on how the selection of immune-resistant phenotypes leads to resistance against cancer immunotherapy:

1. Immune Selection Pressure:
   - Cancer immunotherapy exerts selective pressure on tumors, aiming to target and eliminate tumor cells recognized by the immune system.
   - The immune system's ability to recognize and attack tumor cells creates a selection process favoring the survival and growth of immune-resistant phenotypes.

2. Phenotypic Plasticity:
   - Tumor cells possess inherent plasticity, allowing them to adapt to changing

microenvironments and immune pressures.

- Under the selective pressure of immunotherapy, tumor cells can undergo phenotypic changes to escape immune recognition and destruction.

3. Mechanisms of Immune Resistance:

a. Antigen Loss or Downregulation:

- Immune-resistant phenotypes can downregulate or completely lose the expression of antigens targeted by immune cells.

- This alteration reduces the visibility of tumor cells to immune effectors, hindering their recognition and elimination.

b. Altered Antigen Presentation:

- Immune-resistant phenotypes may exhibit defects in the antigen presentation machinery, impairing the generation and display of tumor-specific antigens.

- Inadequate antigen presentation diminishes the ability of immune cells to mount an effective anti-tumor immune response.

c. Immune Checkpoint Activation:

- Immune-resistant phenotypes can upregulate immune checkpoint molecules, such as PD-L1 or CTLA-4, on their cell surface.

- Increased checkpoint expression inhibits the activation and function of immune cells, dampening the immune response against tumor cells.

d. Alterations in Immunogenicity:
   - Immune-resistant phenotypes can undergo genetic or epigenetic changes that alter their immunogenicity.
   - These changes can reduce the recognition of tumor cells by immune effectors, enabling them to evade immune surveillance.

e. Resistance to Cytotoxicity:
   - Immune-resistant phenotypes may develop mechanisms to resist immune-mediated cytotoxicity.
   - These mechanisms can include upregulation of anti-apoptotic proteins, enhanced DNA repair mechanisms, or increased expression of drug efflux pumps.

4. Implications for Immunotherapy Resistance:
   a. Treatment Failure:
   - Immune-resistant phenotypes persist and thrive, leading to treatment failure and diminished response to immunotherapy.
   - The survival and growth of these resistant phenotypes allow the tumor to evade immune attack and continue to progress.

   b. Disease Recurrence and Metastasis:
   - Immune-resistant phenotypes contribute to disease recurrence and the development of metastases.
   - These phenotypes can disseminate to distant sites and establish secondary tumors, further

complicating treatment and prognosis.

5. Strategies to Overcome Immune-Resistant Phenotypes:

a. Combination Therapies:

- Combining multiple immunotherapeutic approaches, such as immune checkpoint inhibitors, targeted therapies, or immune stimulatory agents, can overcome immune resistance.

- Combination therapies synergistically target different resistance mechanisms and enhance the overall anti-tumor immune response.

b. Personalized Treatment Approaches:

- Comprehensive profiling of tumors can help identify specific immune-resistant phenotypes and the underlying molecular alterations.

- Tailoring treatment strategies based on the identified resistance mechanisms can improve therapeutic outcomes.

c. Immunomodulatory Approaches:

- Novel immunomodulatory strategies, such as the use of oncolytic viruses or immune adjuvants, can enhance the immune response against resistant phenotypes.

- These approaches can promote immune cell infiltration, antigen presentation, and cytotoxicity, improving the effectiveness of immunotherapy.

6. Monitoring and Adaptive Strategies:

a. Regular monitoring of treatment response and disease progression can detect the emergence of immune-resistant phenotypes.

b. Adaptive treatment strategies, including timely modifications to therapy regimens, can be implemented to address resistance and optimize treatment outcomes.

In summary, the selection of immune-resistant phenotypes poses a significant challenge to the success of cancer immunotherapy. Understanding the mechanisms of resistance and employing combination therapies, personalized approaches, and adaptive strategies are crucial for overcoming immune resistance, improving treatment responses, and preventing disease recurrence.

THE EVOLUTIONARY
DYNAMICS WITHIN THE TUMOR
MICROENVIRONMENT

The evolutionary dynamics within the tumor microenvironment play a pivotal role in the development of cancer immunotherapy resistance. As tumors grow and interact with the immune system, a complex interplay occurs between tumor cells, immune cells, and the surrounding microenvironment. This dynamic process can lead to the emergence and selection of resistant phenotypes. Here is a detailed discussion on how the evolutionary dynamics within the tumor microenvironment contribute to cancer immunotherapy resistance:

1. Genetic and Phenotypic Heterogeneity:
   - Tumors exhibit genetic and phenotypic heterogeneity, meaning that they consist of diverse populations of cells with distinct genetic alterations, gene expression profiles, and phenotypes.
   - This heterogeneity provides a basis for evolutionary dynamics within the tumor, as

different cell populations compete and respond differently to selective pressures.

2. Clonal Evolution and Selection:

- Tumors undergo clonal evolution, where genetic alterations and mutations occur over time, leading to the emergence of new subclones.

- These genetic changes can confer advantages to certain tumor cell populations, allowing them to proliferate and survive under selective pressures, such as immune-mediated attack.

3. Immune Selection Pressure:

- Cancer immunotherapy, including immune checkpoint inhibitors and adoptive cell therapies, applies selective pressure on tumor cells by targeting specific antigens or immune checkpoints.

- Immune cells aim to eliminate tumor cells that are recognized as non-self or abnormal.

- However, this immune selection pressure can drive the evolution and selection of tumor cell populations that are less susceptible to immune attack.

4. Immune Editing:

- The interaction between the immune system and tumor cells can lead to a process called immune editing, which consists of three phases: elimination, equilibrium, and escape.

- In the elimination phase, the immune system recognizes and eliminates tumor cells.

- However, during the equilibrium phase, some tumor cells can enter a state of dormancy or undergo genetic changes to evade immune detection.

- Ultimately, in the escape phase, immune-resistant clones emerge and dominate the tumor, leading to immunotherapy resistance.

5. Dynamic Interactions in the Tumor Microenvironment:

- The tumor microenvironment consists of various cell types, including tumor cells, immune cells, stromal cells, and extracellular matrix components.

- Cellular interactions and the release of signaling molecules within the tumor microenvironment shape the evolutionary dynamics.

- For example, immune cells can exert selective pressure on tumor cells, while tumor cells can release factors that promote immunosuppression and create a favorable environment for resistant phenotypes to thrive.

6. Fitness Advantage of Resistant Phenotypes:

- Within the tumor microenvironment, certain phenotypes or subclones may possess inherent or acquired mechanisms that confer resistance to immunotherapy.

- These resistant phenotypes can have a fitness advantage, allowing them to survive and proliferate even in the presence of immune-mediated attack.

- As a result, they outcompete susceptible cell populations, leading to the dominance of resistant clones and immunotherapy resistance.

7. Implications for Immunotherapy Resistance:

- The evolutionary dynamics within the tumor microenvironment have significant implications for cancer immunotherapy resistance:

a. Treatment Failure: The emergence and selection of resistant phenotypes contribute to the failure of immunotherapeutic interventions.

b. Disease Progression: Resistant phenotypes can drive tumor growth, metastasis, and disease progression.

c. Relapse: Even after an initial response to immunotherapy, resistant phenotypes can persist and give rise to disease relapse.

8. Strategies to Overcome Resistance:

- Combining therapies: Combining different immunotherapeutic approaches, such as immune checkpoint inhibitors, targeted therapies, or immunomodulatory agents, can target multiple resistance mechanisms simultaneously and improve treatment outcomes.

- Monitoring and adaptive strategies: Regular monitoring of treatment response and disease progression can help detect the emergence of resistant phenotypes, guiding the adjustment of treatment regimens in a timely manner.

- Personalized medicine: Understanding the

genetic and phenotypic landscape of tumors through comprehensive profiling can aid in the identification of specific resistance mechanisms, enabling the design of personalized treatment strategies.

In conclusion, the evolutionary dynamics within the tumor microenvironment contribute significantly to the development of cancer immunotherapy resistance. The interplay between tumor cells, immune cells, and the surrounding microenvironment drives the selection and dominance of immune-resistant phenotypes. Understanding these dynamics and developing strategies to overcome resistance are critical for improving the effectiveness of cancer immunotherapy and achieving better treatment outcomes.

MUTATION-DRIVEN
RESISTANCE MECHANISMS

Mutation-driven resistance mechanisms are key factors contributing to cancer immunotherapy resistance. Tumor cells can acquire genetic alterations or mutations that enable them to evade immune recognition and elimination. These mutations can occur spontaneously or as a result of selective pressures exerted by the immune system or therapeutic interventions. Here is a detailed discussion on mutation-driven resistance mechanisms leading to cancer immunotherapy resistance:

1. Loss-of-Function Mutations in Antigen Presentation Pathways:

   - Tumor cells can acquire mutations in genes involved in antigen processing and presentation pathways, such as HLA genes or components of the antigen presentation machinery (e.g., TAP1, TAP2, or β2-microglobulin).

   - These loss-of-function mutations impair the ability of tumor cells to present antigens to immune cells, reducing their recognition and targeting by the immune system.

2. Alterations in Tumor Antigens:
- Mutations in genes encoding tumor antigens can result in structural changes or altered antigen expression levels.
- These alterations can reduce the immunogenicity of tumor cells, diminishing their recognition by immune cells and limiting the effectiveness of immunotherapy.

3. Neoantigen Loss or Downregulation:
- Neoantigens, which are antigens derived from tumor-specific mutations, are important targets for immune recognition and response.
- Tumor cells can undergo further genetic mutations that result in the loss or downregulation of neoantigens, evading immune surveillance and reducing the efficacy of immunotherapy.

4. Activation of Immune Checkpoint Pathways:
- Mutations in genes related to immune checkpoints, such as CTLA-4 or PD-L1, can lead to constitutive activation of these pathways.
- Constant activation of immune checkpoint molecules on tumor cells inhibits immune cell activation and dampens the anti-tumor immune response, contributing to immunotherapy resistance.

5. Upregulation of Drug Efflux Pumps:
- Tumor cells can acquire mutations in genes

encoding drug efflux pumps, such as ABC transporters, which actively pump out therapeutic agents from within the cells.

- Increased expression of drug efflux pumps reduces the intracellular concentration of immunotherapeutic drugs, limiting their efficacy and promoting resistance.

6. Activation of Survival Pathways:

- Mutations in genes involved in pro-survival signaling pathways, such as the PI3K-AKT-mTOR pathway, can confer resistance to immune-mediated cell death.

- Activation of these survival pathways promotes tumor cell survival, inhibits apoptosis, and enables evasion of immune attack.

7. Genetic Heterogeneity and Clonal Selection:

- Tumors consist of multiple clonal populations with different genetic alterations.

- Under selective pressure from immunotherapy, certain clones harboring mutations that confer resistance have a survival advantage and can outgrow susceptible clones, leading to immunotherapy resistance.

8. Implications for Immunotherapy Resistance:

- Mutation-driven resistance mechanisms can significantly impact the effectiveness of cancer immunotherapy:

a. Treatment Failure: Mutations that confer resistance can render immunotherapy ineffective, leading to treatment failure.

b. Disease Progression: Resistant clones with genetic alterations can drive tumor growth, invasion, and metastasis.

c. Relapse: Even after an initial response to immunotherapy, resistant clones can survive and give rise to disease relapse.

9. Strategies to Overcome Mutation-Driven Resistance:

- Combination Therapies: Combining immunotherapeutic agents with targeted therapies or other immunomodulatory approaches can target both resistant clones and the tumor microenvironment, improving treatment outcomes.

- Next-Generation Sequencing: Comprehensive genomic profiling and identification of resistance-associated mutations can guide the selection of personalized treatment strategies.

- Rational Drug Design: Understanding the molecular mechanisms underlying resistance can facilitate the development of novel drugs and therapeutic strategies specifically targeting resistance-driving mutations.

In summary, mutation-driven resistance mechanisms play a significant role in cancer immunotherapy resistance. Tumor cells can acquire genetic alterations that confer the ability to evade immune recognition and elimination. Understanding these mechanisms and developing strategies to target and overcome them are crucial for improving the effectiveness of cancer immunotherapy and achieving better treatment outcomes.

ACTIVATION OF BYPASS
SIGNALING PATHWAYS

A ctivation of bypass signaling pathways is a significant mechanism leading to cancer immunotherapy resistance. Tumor cells can activate alternative signaling pathways that circumvent the intended effects of immunotherapy, allowing them to survive and proliferate despite immune attack. Here is a detailed discussion on how the activation of bypass signaling pathways contributes to cancer immunotherapy resistance:

1. Activation of Survival and Proliferation Pathways:
 - Tumor cells can activate alternative survival and proliferation signaling pathways in response to immune-mediated cytotoxicity.
 - For example, activation of the PI3K-AKT-mTOR pathway can promote cell survival, inhibit apoptosis, and facilitate resistance to immune-induced cell death.

2. Activation of Parallel Oncogenic Signaling

Pathways:

- Tumor cells can activate parallel oncogenic signaling pathways that bypass the intended effects of immunotherapy.

- These pathways, such as MAPK/ERK or JAK/STAT signaling, can promote cell growth, survival, and immune evasion, thereby conferring resistance to immunotherapy.

3. Upregulation of Growth Factor Receptors:

- Tumor cells can upregulate the expression of growth factor receptors, such as EGFR, HER2, or MET, as an adaptive response to immune-mediated attack.

- Activation of these receptors can trigger downstream signaling cascades that promote cell survival, proliferation, and resistance to immunotherapy.

4. Activation of Alternative Immune Checkpoint Pathways:

- In addition to well-known immune checkpoints (e.g., PD-L1/PD-1, CTLA-4), tumor cells can activate alternative immune checkpoint molecules or pathways.

- For instance, upregulation of TIM-3, LAG-3, or VISTA can suppress immune responses and contribute to immunotherapy resistance by inhibiting T cell functions.

5. Epithelial-Mesenchymal Transition (EMT):

- The activation of EMT, a cellular program

involved in tissue remodeling and metastasis, can confer resistance to immunotherapy.

- During EMT, tumor cells acquire a mesenchymal phenotype characterized by increased motility, invasiveness, and resistance to immune-mediated cytotoxicity.

6. Activation of DNA Damage Response Pathways:

- Tumor cells can activate DNA damage response pathways in response to immune-mediated cytotoxicity.

- Activation of these pathways can enhance DNA repair mechanisms, allowing tumor cells to survive and resist the effects of immunotherapy.

7. Implications for Immunotherapy Resistance:

- Activation of bypass signaling pathways can have significant implications for cancer immunotherapy resistance:

a. Treatment Failure: Activation of alternative pathways can render immunotherapy ineffective, leading to treatment failure.

b. Immune Evasion: Tumor cells can evade immune recognition and attack by activating alternative survival and immune checkpoint pathways.

c. Disease Progression: Activation of bypass signaling pathways can promote tumor growth, invasion, and metastasis despite ongoing immunotherapy.

8. Strategies to Overcome Bypass Signaling

Pathways:

- Combination Therapies: Combining immunotherapy with targeted inhibitors of alternative signaling pathways can disrupt bypass mechanisms and enhance treatment efficacy.

- Targeted Therapies: Identifying specific genetic alterations and activating mutations driving bypass signaling pathways can guide the selection of targeted therapies to overcome resistance.

- Rational Drug Design: Developing novel drugs that directly target and inhibit key molecules or pathways involved in bypass signaling can prevent or reverse immunotherapy resistance.

In summary, the activation of bypass signaling pathways is a critical mechanism contributing to cancer immunotherapy resistance. Tumor cells can activate alternative survival, proliferation, and immune evasion pathways, allowing them to bypass the intended effects of immunotherapy. Understanding these mechanisms and implementing combination therapies or targeted interventions can help overcome bypass signaling-mediated resistance and improve the effectiveness of cancer immunotherapy.

LOSS OF ANTIGEN PRESENTATION MACHINERY GENES

Loss of antigen presentation machinery genes is a significant mechanism leading to cancer immunotherapy resistance. Antigen presentation is a crucial process for the recognition and elimination of tumor cells by the immune system. However, alterations or mutations in genes involved in antigen presentation pathways can disrupt this process, allowing tumor cells to evade immune surveillance and immunotherapy. Here is a detailed discussion on how the loss of antigen presentation machinery genes contributes to cancer immunotherapy resistance:

1. HLA Class I Genes:
   - Human leukocyte antigen (HLA) class I molecules play a central role in antigen presentation to cytotoxic T cells.
   - Loss-of-function mutations or downregulation of HLA class I genes, such as HLA-A, HLA-B, and HLA-C, can impair the presentation

of tumor antigens to immune cells.

- Without proper antigen presentation, tumor cells become less susceptible to immune recognition and elimination.

2. Beta-2 Microglobulin (β2M):

- β2M is an essential component of HLA class I molecules, required for their proper expression on the cell surface.

- Mutations or deletions in the β2M gene can result in the loss or reduced expression of HLA class I molecules, compromising antigen presentation.

- Tumor cells lacking β2M expression are less likely to be recognized and targeted by cytotoxic T cells.

3. Transporter Associated with Antigen Processing (TAP):

- The TAP complex is responsible for transporting peptides into the endoplasmic reticulum (ER) for loading onto HLA class I molecules.

- Mutations or deficiencies in TAP1 or TAP2 genes can impair peptide transport, leading to a reduced pool of antigenic peptides available for presentation.

- The compromised antigen presentation hinders immune recognition and decreases the effectiveness of immunotherapy.

4. Downregulation of Antigen Processing

Machinery (APM) Components:

- Antigen processing machinery (APM) components, including the proteasome and various chaperones, are involved in antigen processing and presentation.

- Downregulation or mutations in genes encoding APM components, such as LMP2, LMP7, or TAPBP, can disrupt antigen processing and presentation.

- This disruption results in a diminished repertoire of tumor antigens presented to immune cells, limiting their ability to mount an effective antitumor immune response.

5. Impaired Cross-Presentation:

- Cross-presentation is the process by which antigen-presenting cells, such as dendritic cells, present antigens derived from extracellular sources on HLA class I molecules.

- Defects in genes involved in cross-presentation, such as CD74 or LAMP1, can impair the ability of antigen-presenting cells to present tumor antigens effectively.

- Consequently, immune cells may fail to recognize and eliminate tumor cells presenting cross-presented antigens, leading to immunotherapy resistance.

6. Implications for Immunotherapy Resistance:

- Loss of antigen presentation machinery genes can have significant implications for cancer immunotherapy resistance:

a. Immune Escape: Tumor cells lacking proper antigen presentation become less recognizable to immune cells, enabling them to evade immune detection and elimination.

b. Diminished Tumor-specific Immune Response: The reduced presentation of tumor antigens limits the activation and expansion of tumor-specific T cells, hampering the efficacy of immunotherapy.

c. Impaired Immunogenicity: The loss of antigen presentation machinery genes may reduce the immunogenicity of tumor cells, making them less responsive to immunotherapy.

7. Strategies to Overcome Antigen Presentation Machinery Loss:

- Targeted Therapies: Developing targeted therapies that can restore or enhance the expression and function of antigen presentation machinery genes may help overcome resistance

.

- Combination Therapies: Combining immunotherapy with strategies that promote antigen presentation, such as immune modulators or cytokines, can enhance the immune response against tumor cells.

- Adoptive Cell Therapies: Adoptive transfer of genetically modified T cells expressing chimeric antigen receptors (CAR-T cells) can bypass the need for antigen presentation machinery and directly target tumor antigens.

In conclusion, the loss of antigen presentation machinery genes is a significant mechanism leading to cancer immunotherapy resistance. Disruptions in antigen presentation impair the recognition and elimination of tumor cells by the immune system. Understanding these mechanisms and developing strategies to restore or enhance antigen presentation are crucial for improving the effectiveness of cancer immunotherapy and overcoming resistance.

DNA METHYLATION AND HISTONE MODIFICATIONS

DNA methylation and histone modifications are epigenetic alterations that can contribute to cancer immunotherapy resistance. These modifications can affect gene expression patterns, including genes involved in immune response and tumor immunogenicity. Here is a detailed discussion on how DNA methylation and histone modifications can lead to cancer immunotherapy resistance:

1. DNA Methylation:
   - DNA methylation refers to the addition of a methyl group to the DNA molecule, often occurring at cytosine residues within CpG dinucleotides.
   - Hypermethylation of CpG islands, which are regions of high CpG density near gene promoters, can lead to gene silencing.
   - Methylation-mediated gene silencing can impact immune-related genes, including those involved in antigen presentation, immune cell activation, and tumor suppressor genes.

- Hypermethylation of these genes can result in reduced antigen presentation, impaired immune cell function, and dampened antitumor immune response.

2. Histone Modifications:
-    Histone modifications involve various chemical changes to the histone proteins around which DNA is wrapped, influencing chromatin structure and gene expression.
-    Histone modifications can include acetylation, methylation, phosphorylation, and ubiquitination, among others.
- Alterations in histone modifications can affect the accessibility of DNA to the transcriptional machinery, impacting gene expression patterns.
- Dysregulation of histone modifications can lead to the silencing of immune-related genes and the downregulation of tumor antigens, limiting immune recognition and response.

3. Immune Checkpoint Genes:
- DNA methylation and histone modifications can influence the expression of immune checkpoint genes, such as PD-1, PD-L1, and CTLA-4.
- Hypermethylation of immune checkpoint genes or repressive histone modifications at their promoters can lead to reduced expression of these molecules.
- Reduced expression of immune checkpoints can hinder immune regulation and impair the

effectiveness of immunotherapy targeting these pathways.

4. Tumor Antigen Genes:
   - Epigenetic modifications can impact the expression of tumor antigen genes, including those encoding cancer-testis antigens or neoantigens.
   - Hypermethylation or repressive histone modifications at the promoters of these genes can lead to their downregulation or silencing.
   - Reduced expression of tumor antigens diminishes their presentation to immune cells, limiting immune recognition and targeting of tumor cells.

5. Immune Cell Function Genes:
   - Epigenetic alterations can affect genes involved in immune cell activation, function, and effector mechanisms.
   - Hypermethylation or repressive histone modifications in these genes can dampen immune cell responses and impair antitumor immunity.
   - Altered expression of immune cell function genes can reduce the cytotoxicity, proliferation, and cytokine production of immune cells, limiting their effectiveness in eliminating tumor cells.

6. Implications for Immunotherapy Resistance:
   - DNA methylation and histone modifications can have several implications for cancer immunotherapy resistance:

a. Immune Evasion: Epigenetic alterations can contribute to immune evasion by reducing antigen presentation, immune cell activation, and tumor immunogenicity.

b. Diminished Response to Immunotherapy: Hypermethylation or repressive histone modifications can render tumor cells less responsive to immunotherapy by altering the expression of immune checkpoint genes and immune cell function genes.

c. Heterogeneity of Epigenetic Alterations: Epigenetic modifications can exhibit inter-tumor and intra-tumor heterogeneity, further complicating treatment strategies.

7. Strategies to Overcome Epigenetic-Mediated Resistance:

- Epigenetic Modulators: Targeting DNA methylation or histone modifications using epigenetic modulating agents, such as DNA demethylating agents (e.g., azacitidine) or histone deacetylase inhibitors (e.g., vorinostat), can potentially reverse the epigenetic alterations and enhance immunotherapy efficacy.

- Combination Therapies: Combining immunotherapy with epigenetic modulators can synergistically target both the immune system and the underlying epigenetic alterations, improving treatment outcomes.

- Biomarker Development: Identifying specific epigenetic alterations associated with immunotherapy resistance can help in the development of predictive biomarkers for patient stratification and personalized treatment approaches.

In conclusion, DNA methylation and histone modifications can contribute to cancer immunotherapy resistance by impacting gene expression patterns relevant to immune response and tumor immunogenicity. Understanding these epigenetic alterations and developing strategies to reverse or overcome them can enhance the effectiveness of immunotherapy and overcome resistance mechanisms in cancer treatment.

ALTERATIONS IN GENE
EXPRESSION PATTERNS

Alterations in gene expression patterns can play a significant role in cancer immunotherapy resistance. These alterations can affect multiple genes and pathways involved in immune recognition, immune response, and tumor cell behavior. Here is a detailed discussion on how alterations in gene expression patterns can lead to cancer immunotherapy resistance:

1. Downregulation of Antigen Presentation Machinery:

- Altered gene expression can lead to the downregulation of genes involved in antigen processing and presentation, such as HLA class I genes, TAP1/2, or β2M.

- Reduced expression of these genes hinders the presentation of tumor antigens to immune cells, diminishing immune recognition and subsequent antitumor response.

2. Immune Checkpoint Upregulation:

- Altered gene expression patterns can result

in the upregulation of immune checkpoint molecules, such as PD-L1, CTLA-4, or TIM-3.

- Increased expression of these molecules can suppress immune responses, inhibit T cell activation and proliferation, and promote immune tolerance, leading to immunotherapy resistance.

3. Dysregulated Signaling Pathways:

- Alterations in gene expression can lead to dysregulated signaling pathways, such as the PI3K-AKT-mTOR or MAPK/ERK pathways.

- Dysregulation of these pathways can promote cell survival, proliferation, and immune evasion, enabling tumor cells to resist immunotherapy-induced cytotoxicity.

4. Impaired Tumor Antigen Expression:

- Altered gene expression can result in the downregulation or loss of tumor antigen genes, including cancer-testis antigens or neoantigens.

- Reduced expression of tumor antigens limits their presentation to immune cells, reducing immune recognition and targeting of tumor cells.

5. Immunosuppressive Factors Upregulation:

- Gene expression alterations can lead to the upregulation of immunosuppressive factors, such as TGF-β, IL-10, or IDO.

- Increased expression of these factors can create an immunosuppressive tumor microenvironment, inhibiting immune effector functions and promoting immunotherapy resistance.

6. Enhanced DNA Repair Mechanisms:

- Altered gene expression can upregulate DNA repair genes, such as BRCA1/2 or MGMT.

- Enhanced DNA repair capacity allows tumor cells to repair DNA damage induced by immunotherapy, reducing treatment effectiveness and promoting resistance.

7. EMT-Related Gene Expression Changes:

- Epithelial-Mesenchymal Transition (EMT) is associated with altered gene expression patterns that promote tumor cell invasiveness and metastasis.

- EMT-related gene expression changes can contribute to immunotherapy resistance by enabling tumor cells to escape immune recognition and immune attack.

8. Implications for Immunotherapy Resistance:

- Altered gene expression patterns can have several implications for cancer immunotherapy resistance:

a. Reduced Immunogenicity: Downregulation of antigen presentation machinery or tumor antigens decreases the immunogenicity of tumor cells, reducing immune recognition and targeting.

b. Immune Evasion: Upregulation of immune checkpoints or immunosuppressive factors promotes immune evasion and dampens antitumor immune responses.

c. Altered Cell Signaling: Dysregulated signaling pathways and enhanced DNA repair mechanisms provide survival advantages to tumor cells, making them resistant to immunotherapy-induced cytotoxicity.

9. Strategies to Overcome Altered Gene Expression Patterns:

-   Combination Therapies: Combining immunotherapy with targeted therapies or agents that can reverse gene expression alterations may enhance treatment efficacy and overcome resistance.

-   Biomarker Development: Identifying and validating predictive biomarkers associated with altered gene expression patterns can help guide patient selection and treatment decisions.

-   Novel Therapeutic Approaches: Developing innovative therapies targeting specific gene expression alterations, such as gene editing techniques or RNA interference, may offer new strategies to overcome resistance.

In conclusion, alterations in gene expression patterns can contribute to cancer immunotherapy resistance by modulating immune recognition, immune response, and tumor cell behavior. Understanding these alterations and developing strategies to reverse or overcome them are essential for improving the effectiveness of immunotherapy and overcoming resistance mechanisms in cancer treatment.

UPREGULATION OF IMMUNE CHECKPOINT MOLECULES

Upregulation of immune checkpoint molecules is a significant mechanism leading to cancer immunotherapy resistance. Immune checkpoints, such as PD-1, PD-L1, CTLA-4, and TIM-3, play a crucial role in regulating immune responses and maintaining immune homeostasis. Here is a detailed discussion on how upregulation of immune checkpoint molecules can lead to cancer immunotherapy resistance:

1. PD-1/PD-L1 Pathway:
   - Upregulation of PD-1 (programmed cell death protein 1) on T cells and PD-L1 (programmed death-ligand 1) on tumor cells or immune cells is a common mechanism of immune evasion.
   - Increased expression of PD-L1 can engage with PD-1 on T cells, leading to T cell exhaustion, impaired effector functions, and reduced antitumor immune response.
   - Upregulation of PD-L1 can be induced by inflammatory cytokines, oncogenic signaling

pathways, or genetic alterations, contributing to immunotherapy resistance.

2. CTLA-4 Pathway:

- CTLA-4 (cytotoxic T-lymphocyte-associated protein 4) is another immune checkpoint molecule expressed on T cells.

- Upregulation of CTLA-4 can dampen T cell activation and proliferation by outcompeting the co-stimulatory receptor CD28, resulting in decreased antitumor immune response.

- Increased CTLA-4 expression can impair the effectiveness of immunotherapies that target other checkpoints, such as PD-1/PD-L1 inhibitors.

3. TIM-3 Pathway:

- TIM-3 (T cell immunoglobulin and mucin domain-containing protein 3) is an immune checkpoint receptor expressed on T cells and other immune cells.

- Upregulation of TIM-3 can lead to T cell dysfunction, exhaustion, and decreased cytokine production.

- Increased TIM-3 expression has been associated with resistance to immunotherapies, including immune checkpoint blockade therapies.

4. Implications for Immunotherapy Resistance:

- Enhanced Immune Suppression: Upregulation of immune checkpoint molecules creates an immunosuppressive microenvironment, inhibiting effector T cell function and promoting tumor immune evasion.

- Tumor Immune Escape: Increased expression of immune checkpoints allows tumor cells to evade immune surveillance and destruction, contributing to immunotherapy resistance.

- Resistance to Checkpoint Inhibitors: Upregulation of checkpoint molecules can limit the effectiveness of immune checkpoint inhibitors, which aim to block the inhibitory interactions between checkpoint receptors and their ligands.

5. Strategies to Overcome Upregulation of Immune Checkpoint Molecules:

- Combination Therapies: Combining immune checkpoint inhibitors targeting different checkpoint molecules can overcome resistance mediated by upregulation of a specific checkpoint.

- Combination with Targeted Therapies: Combining immunotherapy with targeted therapies that can downregulate immune checkpoint expression or modulate tumor-immune interactions may enhance treatment efficacy.

- Novel Checkpoint Blockade Agents: Developing novel agents targeting upregulated immune checkpoints or co-inhibitory receptors can expand the therapeutic options for resistant tumors.

- Biomarker Development: Identifying predictive biomarkers associated with upregulation of specific immune checkpoints can aid in patient selection and personalized treatment strategies.

In conclusion, upregulation of immune checkpoint molecules, such as PD-1, PD-L1, CTLA-4, and TIM-3, is a key mechanism leading to cancer immunotherapy resistance. Understanding these upregulation mechanisms and developing strategies to overcome checkpoint-mediated immune suppression are crucial for improving the effectiveness of immunotherapy and overcoming resistance in cancer treatment.

RECRUITMENT OF SUPPRESSIVE IMMUNE CELLS

The recruitment of suppressive immune cells into the tumor microenvironment is a significant mechanism contributing to cancer immunotherapy resistance. These suppressive immune cells can create an immunosuppressive milieu that inhibits the function of effector immune cells and promotes tumor growth and immune evasion. Here is a detailed discussion on how the recruitment of suppressive immune cells can lead to cancer immunotherapy resistance:

1. Regulatory T cells (Tregs):
   - Tregs are a subset of CD4+ T cells with immunosuppressive properties.
   - Tumor-infiltrating Tregs can suppress the activity of effector T cells, inhibit antitumor immune responses, and promote immune tolerance.
   - Increased recruitment and accumulation of Tregs within the tumor microenvironment can create an immunosuppressive barrier, limiting the

effectiveness of immunotherapy.

2. Myeloid-Derived Suppressor Cells (MDSCs):

- MDSCs are a heterogeneous population of immature myeloid cells with potent immunosuppressive functions.
- MDSCs can suppress T cell activity, promote T cell exhaustion, and inhibit immune responses against tumors.
- Increased recruitment and accumulation of MDSCs within the tumor microenvironment contribute to immunosuppression and resistance to immunotherapy.

3. Tumor-Associated Macrophages (TAMs):

- TAMs are a type of macrophage that can display immunosuppressive properties.
- They can suppress T cell function, promote angiogenesis, and remodel the tumor microenvironment in favor of tumor growth.
- Enhanced recruitment and polarization of TAMs towards an immunosuppressive phenotype can hinder immune responses and confer resistance to immunotherapy.

4. M2 Macrophages:

- M2 macrophages are a subset of macrophages with immunosuppressive and tissue remodeling functions.
- They can inhibit T cell responses, promote tumor angiogenesis, and contribute to tumor immune escape.

- Increased recruitment and polarization of M2 macrophages within the tumor microenvironment contribute to immunosuppression and immunotherapy resistance.

5. Neutrophils:

- Neutrophils are the most abundant type of white blood cells and can exhibit both pro- and anti-tumor properties.

- Some subsets of neutrophils, such as tumor-associated neutrophils (TANs) with an immunosuppressive phenotype, can suppress T cell responses and promote tumor progression.

- Enhanced recruitment of immunosuppressive neutrophils can impair immune responses and contribute to immunotherapy resistance.

6. Implications for Immunotherapy Resistance:

- Immunosuppressive Microenvironment: The recruitment of suppressive immune cells creates an immunosuppressive microenvironment that inhibits the function of effector immune cells and promotes tumor growth and immune evasion.

- Inhibition of Antitumor Immune Responses: Suppressive immune cells can directly inhibit the activity of cytotoxic T cells, NK cells, and other immune effector cells, limiting their ability to target and eliminate tumor cells.

- Altered Cytokine Milieu: The presence of suppressive immune cells can lead to the secretion of immunosuppressive cytokines and factors that further dampen antitumor immune responses.

7. Strategies to Overcome Suppressive Immune Cell Recruitment:

- Targeted Depletion: Therapeutic strategies targeting suppressive immune cells, such as Tregs or MDSCs, can be used to reduce their abundance and restore antitumor immune responses.

- Repolarization of Immune Cells: Modulating the polarization of TAMs and neutrophils from an immunosuppressive to an immunostimulatory phenotype can enhance immune responses and overcome resistance.

- Combination Therapies: Combining immunotherapy with agents that target suppressive immune cells or their recruitment factors can synergistically enhance treatment efficacy.

In conclusion, the recruitment of suppressive immune cells into the tumor microenvironment is a key mechanism leading to cancer immunotherapy resistance. Understanding the interactions between these cells and the tumor microenvironment and developing strategies to overcome their immunosuppressive effects are essential for improving the effectiveness of immunotherapy and overcoming resistance in cancer treatment.

MODULATION OF THE TUMOR MICROENVIRONMENT

Modulation of the tumor microenvironment is a critical factor contributing to cancer immunotherapy resistance. The tumor microenvironment is a complex ecosystem consisting of various cell types, extracellular matrix components, signaling molecules, and immune cells. Alterations within the tumor microenvironment can create an immunosuppressive and protumorigenic milieu that hinders effective antitumor immune responses. Here is a detailed discussion on how the modulation of the tumor microenvironment can lead to cancer immunotherapy resistance:

1. Immunosuppressive Factors:
   - The tumor microenvironment can produce immunosuppressive factors such as TGF-β, IL-10, adenosine, and prostaglandins.
   - These factors can inhibit T cell activation and proliferation, induce T cell exhaustion, and promote the expansion of regulatory T cells and myeloid-derived suppressor cells.

- Increased production of immunosuppressive factors within the tumor microenvironment contributes to immune evasion and resistance to immunotherapy.

2. Stromal Cells and Extracellular Matrix (ECM):

- Cancer-associated fibroblasts (CAFs) and other stromal cells in the tumor microenvironment can promote immunosuppression and tissue remodeling.

- CAFs can secrete factors that inhibit immune cell function and remodel the ECM, creating physical barriers for immune cell infiltration.

- The dense ECM can limit the penetration of immune cells and therapeutic agents into the tumor, hindering treatment efficacy.

3. Angiogenesis and Hypoxia:

- Tumor angiogenesis, the formation of new blood vessels, is often dysregulated within the tumor microenvironment.

- Abnormal blood vessel formation can lead to hypoxia (low oxygen levels) within the tumor, which further promotes immunosuppression and resistance to therapy.

- Hypoxic conditions can upregulate the expression of immunosuppressive molecules and induce the recruitment of suppressive immune cells.

4. Metabolic Reprogramming:

- Tumor cells often undergo metabolic

reprogramming, resulting in increased nutrient uptake and altered metabolic pathways.

- Metabolic changes within the tumor microenvironment can create an immunosuppressive milieu by limiting the availability of nutrients and generating metabolic byproducts that suppress immune responses.

- Metabolic competition between tumor cells and immune cells can impair immune cell function and contribute to immunotherapy resistance.

5. Genetic and Epigenetic Alterations:

- Genetic mutations and epigenetic modifications can occur within both tumor cells and cells of the tumor microenvironment.

- These alterations can lead to dysregulated signaling pathways, immune evasion mechanisms, and altered cytokine profiles, promoting immunosuppression and resistance to immunotherapy.

6. Implications for Immunotherapy Resistance:

- Immune Exclusion: Modulation of the tumor microenvironment can lead to the exclusion of immune cells from the tumor, limiting their ability to recognize and eliminate tumor cells.

- Immune Suppression: The immunosuppressive microenvironment can inhibit immune cell activation, induce T cell dysfunction and exhaustion, and dampen antitumor immune responses.

- Altered Signaling and Communication: Dysregulated signaling within the tumor microenvironment can interfere with immune cell communication and compromise the effectiveness of immunotherapy.

7. Strategies to Modulate the Tumor Microenvironment:

- Combination Therapies: Combining immunotherapy with agents targeting the tumor microenvironment, such as angiogenesis inhibitors or stroma-modulating agents, may enhance treatment efficacy.

- Targeting Immunomodulatory Factors: Therapeutic interventions targeting immunosuppressive factors, such as cytokine inhibitors or metabolic inhibitors, can overcome immunosuppression and improve immunotherapy outcomes.

- Immune Cell Activation: Strategies aimed at stimulating immune cell activation, such as cytokine administration or immune agonists,

can enhance antitumor immune responses despite the immunosuppressive microenvironment.

- Modulating Hypoxia and Angiogenesis: Agents targeting tumor angiogenesis or hypoxic signaling pathways can normalize the tumor microenvironment and improve immune cell infiltration and function.

In conclusion, the modulation of the

tumor microenvironment is a critical factor leading to cancer immunotherapy resistance. Understanding the complex interactions and mechanisms within the tumor microenvironment and developing strategies to modulate its immunosuppressive properties are essential for overcoming resistance and improving the effectiveness of immunotherapy in cancer treatment.

DUAL IMMUNE CHECKPOINT BLOCKADE

D ual immune checkpoint blockade refers to the simultaneous targeting of two immune checkpoint molecules with blocking antibodies to enhance the antitumor immune response and overcome resistance to cancer immunotherapy. Here is a detailed discussion on the concept and potential benefits of dual immune checkpoint blockade:

1. Immune Checkpoint Blockade:
  - Immune checkpoint molecules, such as PD-1, PD-L1, CTLA-4, and TIM-3, play a crucial role in regulating immune responses and maintaining immune homeostasis.
  - Blockade of immune checkpoints using monoclonal antibodies can release the brakes on the immune system, allowing for enhanced activation and proliferation of effector T cells and improved antitumor immune responses.

2. Mechanism of Dual Immune Checkpoint Blockade:
  - Dual immune checkpoint blockade involves

the simultaneous targeting of two immune checkpoint molecules with blocking antibodies.

- By blocking multiple immune checkpoints, this approach aims to overcome resistance mechanisms and enhance the antitumor immune response synergistically.

3. Complementary Mechanisms:
- Different immune checkpoint molecules operate through distinct signaling pathways and have complementary roles in regulating immune responses.

- Dual blockade can target multiple inhibitory pathways simultaneously, resulting in more comprehensive inhibition of immunosuppressive signals and increased activation of effector T cells.

4. Enhanced T Cell Activation and Function:
- Dual immune checkpoint blockade can lead to enhanced activation and function of T cells within the tumor microenvironment.

- By blocking multiple inhibitory pathways, the therapy can restore T cell effector functions, such as cytokine production, cytotoxicity, and proliferation, resulting in improved antitumor immune responses.

5. Overcoming Resistance Mechanisms:
- Resistance to single checkpoint blockade therapy can occur due to various mechanisms, including upregulation of alternative immune checkpoints, recruitment of suppressive immune

cells, and alterations in antigen presentation.

- Dual immune checkpoint blockade can target multiple resistance mechanisms simultaneously, offering a more comprehensive approach to overcome resistance and improve treatment outcomes.

6. Clinical Efficacy:

- Dual immune checkpoint blockade has shown promising results in preclinical and clinical studies.

- Combination therapies, such as anti-PD-1/PD-L1 plus anti-CTLA-4 antibodies, have demonstrated enhanced response rates and improved overall survival compared to single checkpoint blockade in certain cancer types, such as melanoma and lung cancer.

7. Safety Considerations:

- Dual immune checkpoint blockade can lead to increased immune-related adverse events (irAEs) compared to monotherapy.

- Close monitoring and management of irAEs are crucial to ensure the safety and well-being of patients receiving dual checkpoint blockade therapy.

8. Future Directions:

- Identifying predictive biomarkers that can guide the selection of patients who are more likely to benefit from dual checkpoint blockade is an active area of research.

- Exploring novel combinations and sequencing strategies with other immunotherapies, targeted agents, or conventional treatments may further optimize the therapeutic outcomes.

In conclusion, dual immune checkpoint blockade represents a promising approach to overcome resistance to cancer immunotherapy. By simultaneously targeting multiple immune checkpoints, this strategy aims to enhance T cell activation, overcome resistance mechanisms, and improve treatment responses. Continued research and clinical trials will provide further insights into the optimal combinations, patient selection, and management of adverse events associated with dual immune checkpoint blockade therapy.

COMBINING IMMUNE CHECKPOINT INHIBITORS

Combining immune checkpoint inhibitors with targeted therapies is an emerging approach aimed at overcoming resistance to cancer immunotherapy. This strategy leverages the complementary mechanisms of immune checkpoint inhibitors and targeted therapies to enhance antitumor immune responses and improve treatment outcomes. Here is a detailed discussion on the concept and potential benefits of combining immune checkpoint inhibitors with targeted therapies:

1. Immune Checkpoint Inhibitors:

- Immune checkpoint inhibitors, such as anti-PD-1, anti-PD-L1, and anti-CTLA-4 antibodies, block inhibitory signals in the immune system, allowing for enhanced activation and proliferation of effector T cells.

- Immune checkpoint inhibitors have demonstrated remarkable clinical efficacy in certain cancer types, leading to durable responses and improved overall survival.

2. Targeted Therapies:

- Targeted therapies specifically inhibit molecular targets that drive tumor growth, survival, or angiogenesis.

- These therapies often target specific genetic alterations or dysregulated signaling pathways present in cancer cells.

- Targeted therapies have shown significant clinical benefits in patients with specific genetic alterations or molecular subtypes of cancer.

3. Complementary Mechanisms:

- Immune checkpoint inhibitors and targeted therapies operate through distinct mechanisms of action and can have complementary effects on the tumor microenvironment.

- Targeted therapies can modulate tumor cells, alter the expression of immune checkpoint molecules, and affect antigen presentation, making the tumor more susceptible to immune attack.

- Immune checkpoint inhibitors can unleash the full potential of the immune system, enhancing antitumor immune responses and promoting the eradication of targeted therapy-treated tumor cells.

4. Overcoming Resistance Mechanisms:

- Resistance to targeted therapies can occur through various mechanisms, such as the emergence of secondary mutations or activation of alternative signaling pathways.

- Immune checkpoint inhibitors can overcome resistance mechanisms by activating antitumor immune responses, targeting the immune-evading properties of tumor cells, and promoting immune-mediated tumor cell death.

5. Synergistic Effects:

- The combination of immune checkpoint inhibitors and targeted therapies can lead to synergistic effects, resulting in improved treatment outcomes.

- Targeted therapies can sensitize tumor cells to immune recognition and enhance the immunogenicity of the tumor, making it more responsive to immune checkpoint blockade.

- Immune checkpoint inhibitors can potentiate the effects of targeted therapies by activating immune cells, increasing tumor infiltration, and promoting durable immune memory responses.

6. Clinical Efficacy:

- Preclinical and clinical studies have demonstrated the potential benefits of combining immune checkpoint inhibitors with targeted therapies in various cancer types.

- For example, combining immune checkpoint inhibitors with targeted therapies, such as BRAF or MEK inhibitors in melanoma, has shown improved response rates and prolonged survival compared to monotherapy.

7. Personalized Approaches:

- The selection of appropriate targeted therapies and immune checkpoint inhibitors may be guided by the genetic profile of the tumor, including actionable mutations or alterations.

- Biomarkers, such as tumor mutation burden or immune-related gene expression profiles, may help identify patients who are more likely to benefit from the combination approach.

8. Future Directions:

- Further research is needed to identify optimal combinations, treatment sequences, and dosing regimens for immune checkpoint inhibitors and targeted therapies.

- Biomarker discovery and validation are crucial for patient selection and identifying predictive markers of response to combination therapies.

- Ongoing clinical trials are evaluating the efficacy and safety of various combinations, and the results will provide valuable insights into the optimal use of immune checkpoint inhibitors with targeted therapies.

In conclusion, combining immune checkpoint inhibitors with targeted therapies holds great promise for overcoming resistance to cancer immunotherapy. The synergistic effects of these approaches can enhance antitumor immune responses, overcome resistance mechanisms, and improve treatment outcomes for patients with cancer. Continued research and clinical trials

will further refine and optimize the use of combination therapies, ultimately benefiting patients by providing more effective and personalized treatment options.

COMBINING IMMUNOTHERAPY WITH OTHER TREATMENT MODALITIES

Combining immunotherapy with other treatment modalities, such as chemotherapy and radiation, is an active area of research aimed at overcoming resistance to cancer immunotherapy. This multi-modal approach takes advantage of the complementary mechanisms of action of different treatments to enhance antitumor immune responses and improve treatment outcomes. Here is a detailed discussion on the concept and potential benefits of combining immunotherapy with chemotherapy and radiation:

1. Immunotherapy:
-    Immunotherapy, including immune checkpoint inhibitors, adoptive cell therapies, and cancer vaccines, harnesses the power of the immune system to recognize and eliminate cancer cells.
-    Immunotherapy has shown remarkable clinical efficacy in various cancers, leading to

durable responses and improved survival rates.

2. Chemotherapy:
- Chemotherapy involves the use of cytotoxic drugs to kill rapidly dividing cancer cells.

- Chemotherapy agents can have direct cytotoxic effects on tumor cells and induce immunogenic cell death, leading to the release of tumor antigens and activation of immune responses.

- Additionally, chemotherapy can modulate the tumor microenvironment, making it more receptive to immune cell infiltration and immunotherapy.

3. Radiation Therapy:
- Radiation therapy uses high-energy radiation to kill cancer cells and shrink tumors.

- Radiation therapy can induce immunogenic cell death, release tumor antigens, and enhance tumor antigen presentation.

- It can also promote the recruitment of immune cells into the tumor microenvironment and modulate the immunosuppressive properties of the tumor, making it more amenable to immunotherapy.

4. Synergistic Effects:
- The combination of immunotherapy with chemotherapy or radiation can lead to synergistic effects, resulting in enhanced antitumor immune responses and improved treatment outcomes.

- Chemotherapy and radiation can increase the release of tumor antigens and promote the expression of immune-stimulatory molecules, making the tumor more visible to the immune system.

- Immunotherapy, in turn, can augment the immune response, activate effector immune cells, and overcome immunosuppressive mechanisms, leading to enhanced tumor cell killing.

5. Overcoming Resistance Mechanisms:

- Resistance to immunotherapy can occur due to various mechanisms, such as low tumor mutational burden, immune evasion, or immunosuppressive tumor microenvironment.

- Chemotherapy and radiation can sensitize tumor cells to immune recognition, increase tumor antigenicity, and reverse immunosuppression, addressing some of the resistance mechanisms and improving the effectiveness of immunotherapy.

6. Sequential or Concurrent Approaches:

- The combination of immunotherapy with chemotherapy or radiation can be administered sequentially or concurrently, depending on the specific cancer type, stage, and treatment goals.

- Sequential approaches involve administering one modality followed by the other, taking advantage of the immunomodulatory effects induced by the initial treatment.

- Concurrent approaches involve simultaneous

administration of immunotherapy with chemotherapy or radiation, aiming to synergize their effects and maximize treatment efficacy.

7. Clinical Efficacy:

- Several clinical studies have demonstrated the potential benefits of combining immunotherapy with chemotherapy or radiation in various cancer types, such as lung cancer, melanoma, and bladder cancer.

- Combination regimens have shown improved response rates, prolonged survival, and increased durability of responses compared to monotherapy.

8. Future Directions:

- Further research is needed to optimize the sequencing, dosing, and scheduling of combined treatments to achieve the best therapeutic outcomes.

- Identifying predictive biomarkers that can guide patient selection and predict response to combination therapy is crucial.

- Ongoing clinical trials are exploring different combination approaches and novel treatment regimens, and their results will provide valuable insights into the optimal integration of immunotherapy with chemotherapy and radiation.

In conclusion, combining immunotherapy with chemotherapy or radiation offers a promising approach to overcome resistance and enhance treatment outcomes in cancer patients. The synergistic effects of these modalities, including the release of tumor antigens, modulation of the tumor microenvironment, and activation of immune responses, can improve the effectiveness of immunotherapy. Continued research and clinical trials will further refine and optimize the use of combination regimens, ultimately benefiting patients by providing more effective and personalized treatment strategies.

IDENTIFYING PREDICTIVE BIOMARKERS OF RESPONSE

Identifying predictive biomarkers of response to cancer immunotherapy is crucial for overcoming resistance and optimizing treatment outcomes. These biomarkers can help guide patient selection, predict response to immunotherapy, and enable personalized treatment approaches. Here is a discussion on the importance of predictive biomarkers and some examples of biomarkers currently being investigated:

1. Importance of Predictive Biomarkers:

   - Response to immunotherapy can vary among patients, and not all individuals benefit equally from treatment.

   - Predictive biomarkers help identify patients who are more likely to respond to immunotherapy, sparing non-responders from potential side effects and enabling the use of alternative treatment strategies.

   - Biomarkers can also provide insights into the underlying mechanisms of resistance, facilitating the development of novel therapeutic approaches.

2. Tumor Mutational Burden (TMB):

- TMB refers to the total number of mutations in the tumor genome and is associated with higher immunogenicity.

- High TMB has been shown to correlate with increased response to immune checkpoint inhibitors across multiple cancer types, including lung cancer, melanoma, and bladder cancer.

- TMB is measured through genomic sequencing and can serve as a predictive biomarker for immunotherapy response.

3. Microsatellite Instability (MSI) and DNA Mismatch Repair Deficiency (dMMR):

- MSI and dMMR are markers of defective DNA repair mechanisms, resulting in genomic instability.

- Tumors with MSI or dMMR are more likely to be responsive to immune checkpoint inhibitors.

- These biomarkers have been particularly successful in predicting response in colorectal cancer and some other solid tumor types.

4. Programmed Death-Ligand 1 (PD-L1) Expression:

- PD-L1 is an immune checkpoint molecule expressed on tumor cells and immune cells.

- PD-L1 expression levels have been used as a biomarker for response to PD-1/PD-L1 inhibitors in several cancer types, including lung cancer and bladder cancer.

- However, the utility of PD-L1 expression as a predictive biomarker is still evolving, and its correlation with response is not absolute.

5. Immune Infiltrate and Tumor-Infiltrating Lymphocytes (TILs):

- The presence of a high density of TILs within the tumor microenvironment is associated with improved response to immunotherapy.

- Immune cell infiltrate, such as CD8+ T cells, has been correlated with better clinical outcomes in various cancer types.

- Assessment of immune infiltrate and TILs through histopathological examination or immune profiling techniques can provide valuable predictive information.

6. Genomic Alterations and Neoantigens:

- Specific genomic alterations, such as gene mutations or amplifications, can result in the generation of neoantigens that are recognized by the immune system.

- The presence of neoantigens and their recognition by T cells have been associated with improved response to immunotherapy.

- High-throughput sequencing and bioinformatics approaches are used to identify neoantigens and predict immunogenicity.

7. Other Biomarkers:

- Several other biomarkers, such as immune

gene expression signatures, cytokine profiles, and immune cell subsets, are being investigated for their predictive value.

- Biomarkers related to immune evasion mechanisms, such as regulatory T cells or myeloid-derived suppressor cells, are also under investigation.

8. Combination Biomarkers:

- It is likely that a combination of biomarkers will provide more accurate predictions of response to immunotherapy.

- Biomarker panels or signatures that incorporate multiple factors, such as TMB, PD-L1 expression, and immune cell profiling, are being explored to improve predictive accuracy.

In conclusion, identifying predictive biomarkers of response to cancer immunotherapy is essential for optimizing treatment strategies and overcoming resistance. TMB, MSI/dMMR, PD-L1 expression, immune infiltrate, genomic alterations, and neoantigens are among the biomarkers currently being investigated. As research advances, a comprehensive understanding of these biomarkers and their predictive value will facilitate personalized and effective immunotherapy for patients with cancer.

TAILORING TREATMENT STRATEGIES BASED ON INDIVIDUAL PATIENT CHARACTERISTICS

Tailoring treatment strategies based on individual patient characteristics is a key approach for overcoming resistance to cancer immunotherapy. By considering factors such as tumor biology, immune profile, and genetic makeup, personalized treatment plans can be developed to maximize therapeutic efficacy. Here is a discussion on the importance of individualized treatment strategies and some examples of how different patient characteristics can guide decision-making:

1. Tumor Molecular Profiling:
   - Tumor molecular profiling, such as genomic sequencing, can identify specific genetic alterations and mutations within a tumor.
   - This information can help identify targetable driver mutations and guide the selection of targeted therapies or combination treatment regimens.

- Molecular profiling can also reveal tumor-specific antigens and neoantigens, which may guide the use of immunotherapies such as immune checkpoint inhibitors or personalized cancer vaccines.

2. Immune Profile:

- Assessing the immune profile of a patient can provide insights into the immune system's ability to recognize and eliminate cancer cells.

- Biomarkers such as PD-L1 expression, tumor-infiltrating lymphocytes (TILs), and immune cell subsets can help predict response to immune checkpoint inhibitors.

- Immune profiling can guide the decision to use single-agent immunotherapy or combination approaches, as well as identify potential resistance mechanisms.

3. Biomarkers of Resistance:

- Understanding the underlying mechanisms of resistance to immunotherapy is crucial for tailoring treatment strategies.

- Biomarkers, such as loss of antigen presentation machinery, upregulation of immune checkpoint molecules, or presence of inhibitory immune cells, can guide the selection of combination therapies targeting specific resistance pathways.

- Biomarker-driven approaches can help overcome resistance and improve treatment outcomes.

4. Treatment Sequencing and Combinations:

- Tailoring treatment strategies also involves determining the optimal sequencing and combination of therapies.

- For example, in tumors with high tumor mutational burden or neoantigen expression, starting with immune checkpoint inhibitors may be preferred.

- Sequential or concurrent use of immunotherapy with other modalities, such as chemotherapy or radiation, can enhance antitumor immune responses and overcome resistance mechanisms.

5. Patient-specific Factors:

- Patient-specific factors, including age, performance status, comorbidities, and treatment preferences, should be considered when tailoring treatment strategies.

- Individual patient characteristics may influence treatment tolerability, response rates, and potential toxicities.

- Shared decision-making between patients and healthcare providers is crucial to develop personalized treatment plans that align with patients' goals and preferences.

6. Adaptive Therapy Approaches:

- Adaptive therapy approaches involve dynamically adjusting treatment based on the evolving tumor characteristics and treatment response.

- Regular monitoring of tumor response, biomarkers, and the immune microenvironment can guide treatment adaptations, such as dose modifications, treatment breaks, or switching to alternative therapies.

- Adaptive strategies aim to optimize treatment efficacy while minimizing the development of resistance.

7. Clinical Trials and Research:

- Participating in clinical trials provides access to novel therapies and personalized treatment approaches.

- Clinical trials often incorporate biomarker-driven strategies and offer the opportunity to evaluate new combinations, sequencing, and predictive biomarkers.

- Ongoing research efforts continue to refine our understanding of individual patient characteristics and their impact on treatment response and resistance mechanisms.

In conclusion, tailoring treatment strategies based on individual patient characteristics is essential for overcoming resistance to cancer immunotherapy. Considering tumor molecular profiling, immune profile, biomarkers of resistance, treatment sequencing, patient-specific factors, and adaptive therapy approaches can optimize treatment outcomes and improve patient care. The continued integration of personalized medicine approaches and participation in clinical trials will further advance our ability to overcome resistance and achieve better outcomes for patients receiving immunotherapy.

TARGETING ALTERNATIVE IMMUNE CHECKPOINT PATHWAYS

Targeting alternative immune checkpoint pathways is a promising strategy for overcoming resistance to cancer immunotherapy. While immune checkpoint inhibitors targeting programmed cell death protein 1 (PD-1) or cytotoxic T lymphocyte-associated antigen 4 (CTLA-4) have shown significant clinical benefits in some patients, not all individuals respond to these therapies. Here is a discussion on alternative immune checkpoint pathways and their potential as therapeutic targets:

1. LAG-3 (Lymphocyte Activation Gene-3):

   - LAG-3 is an immune checkpoint molecule expressed on activated T cells and regulatory T cells (Tregs).

   - It plays a role in regulating T cell function and immune tolerance.

   - LAG-3 can suppress T cell responses and promote T cell exhaustion.

- Combining anti-LAG-3 antibodies with PD-1/PD-L1 inhibitors has shown promise in preclinical and clinical studies, with improved antitumor activity observed in certain cancer types.

2. TIM-3 (T cell Immunoglobulin and Mucin domain-containing protein 3):

- TIM-3 is another immune checkpoint molecule expressed on T cells, natural killer cells, and dendritic cells.

- It regulates T cell exhaustion and immune tolerance.

- TIM-3 can negatively regulate T cell function and promote immunosuppression within the tumor microenvironment.

- Dual blockade of TIM-3 and PD-1/PD-L1 has demonstrated synergistic effects in preclinical models and is being evaluated in clinical trials.

3. TIGIT (T cell Immunoreceptor with Ig and ITIM domains):

- TIGIT is an inhibitory receptor expressed on T cells and natural killer cells.

- It competes with the co-stimulatory receptor CD226 (DNAM-1) for binding to shared ligands.

- TIGIT signaling can inhibit T cell activation and promote immune evasion.

- Combined blockade of TIGIT and PD-1/PD-L1 has shown enhanced antitumor immune responses in preclinical models and is under investigation in clinical trials.

4. VISTA (V-domain Ig suppressor of T cell activation):

- VISTA is an immune checkpoint protein expressed on various immune cells, including T cells and antigen-presenting cells.
- It negatively regulates T cell responses and promotes immune suppression.
- Preclinical studies have shown that targeting VISTA in combination with PD-1/PD-L1 blockade enhances antitumor immune responses and improves therapeutic outcomes.

5. B7-H3 (also known as CD276):

- B7-H3 is a cell surface protein expressed on tumor cells and immune cells.
- It has immunomodulatory functions and can inhibit T cell responses.
- Targeting B7-H3 in combination with immune checkpoint inhibitors has demonstrated enhanced antitumor effects in preclinical models and is being evaluated in clinical trials.

6. IDO (Indoleamine 2,3-dioxygenase):

- IDO is an enzyme involved in tryptophan metabolism, which suppresses T cell responses and promotes immune tolerance.
- Inhibition of IDO in combination with immune checkpoint blockade has shown promising results in preclinical studies and is being investigated in clinical trials.

7. Additional Pathways:

- Other immune checkpoint molecules, such as BTLA, CD39, and CD73, are also being explored as potential targets for combination immunotherapy.

- Modulating these pathways in combination with PD-1/PD-L1 or CTLA-4 blockade may enhance the immune response and overcome resistance.

Targeting alternative immune checkpoint pathways provides an opportunity to engage different mechanisms of immune regulation and overcome resistance to traditional immune checkpoint inhibitors. Preclinical and early clinical data suggest that combination therapies targeting multiple checkpoints can lead to improved response rates and better outcomes in certain patient populations. However, further research and clinical trials are needed to fully understand the efficacy and safety of targeting these alternative immune checkpoint pathways and to identify the patient subgroups that are most likely to benefit from such strategies.

ENHANCING T CELL FUNCTION AND ACTIVATION

Enhancing T cell function and activation is a crucial strategy for overcoming resistance to cancer immunotherapy. T cells play a central role in the antitumor immune response, and their dysfunction or exhaustion can contribute to immunotherapy resistance. Here are some approaches to enhance T cell function and activation:

1. Combination Immunotherapies:
   - Combining immune checkpoint inhibitors: Dual blockade of immune checkpoint molecules, such as PD-1 and CTLA-4, can enhance T cell activation and overcome resistance.
   - Combination with targeted therapies: Concurrent or sequential use of targeted therapies, such as tyrosine kinase inhibitors or PARP inhibitors, can enhance T cell responses and improve treatment outcomes.

2. Tumor-Infiltrating Lymphocyte (TIL) Therapy:
   - TIL therapy involves isolating T cells from tumor tissue, expanding them in the laboratory,

and re-infusing them into the patient.

- TILs are enriched with tumor-specific T cells, which can enhance antitumor immune responses.

- TIL therapy has shown promising results in some cancers, particularly melanoma, and ongoing research aims to optimize its effectiveness.

3. Chimeric Antigen Receptor (CAR) T Cell Therapy:

- CAR T cell therapy involves genetically modifying a patient's T cells to express a receptor specific to a tumor antigen.

- CAR T cells can recognize and kill tumor cells in a targeted manner, leading to potent antitumor responses.

- CAR T cell therapy has demonstrated remarkable success in hematological malignancies and is being investigated for solid tumors.

4. T Cell Engagers and Bispecific Antibodies:

- T cell engagers are antibodies designed to bridge T cells and tumor cells, enhancing T cell activation and killing of cancer cells.

- Bispecific antibodies can simultaneously bind to a tumor antigen and an immune cell receptor, promoting T cell activation and tumor cell destruction.

- These approaches can redirect T cells to tumor cells, bypassing immune evasion mechanisms and enhancing antitumor immune responses.

5. Cytokine Therapy:

- Cytokines, such as interleukin-2 (IL-2) and interferons, can promote T cell proliferation, activation, and effector function.

- Administration of cytokines can enhance T cell responses and improve immunotherapy outcomes in selected patients.

6. Metabolic Modulation:

- Modulating the metabolic pathways in T cells can enhance their function and survival.

- Targeting metabolic checkpoints, such as the inhibition of indoleamine 2,3-dioxygenase (IDO) or adenosine signaling, can enhance T cell activation and antitumor responses.

7. Adoptive T Cell Transfer:

- Adoptive T cell transfer involves infusing ex vivo expanded autologous T cells, genetically modified or unmodified, back into the patient.

- This approach can introduce tumor-specific T cells or T cells engineered with tumor-targeting receptors into the patient's immune system to enhance antitumor immunity.

8. Vaccines and Immune Priming:

- Therapeutic cancer vaccines can stimulate the immune system to recognize and target tumor-specific antigens.

- Vaccines can enhance T cell priming and activation, improving the efficacy of subsequent immunotherapies.

9. Immune Modulators:

- Modulating the immune microenvironment using immune modulators, such as toll-like receptor agonists or STING agonists, can enhance T cell activation and overcome immunosuppression.

10. Novel Therapies and Targets:

- Ongoing research is focused on identifying novel targets and developing innovative therapies to enhance T cell function, including next-generation CAR T cells, bi-specific antibodies, and novel immune checkpoint inhibitors.

Enhancing T cell function and activation is a multifaceted approach involving combinations of therapies, immune modulators, and novel treatment strategies. By bolstering T cell responses, overcoming immunosuppression, and promoting tumor recognition and killing, we can improve the efficacy of cancer immunotherapy and overcome resistance. Continued research and clinical trials are essential to refine these approaches and identify the patients who will benefit most from T cell-focused interventions.

IMPROVING ANTIGEN PRESENTATION AND RECOGNITION

Improving antigen presentation and recognition is a crucial aspect of overcoming resistance to cancer immunotherapy. It involves enhancing the ability of tumor cells to present antigens to immune cells and promoting effective recognition of tumor-specific antigens. Here are some strategies aimed at improving antigen presentation and recognition:

1. HLA Expression Modulation:
   - Human leukocyte antigen (HLA) molecules are responsible for presenting antigens to T cells.
   - Enhancing the expression of HLA molecules on tumor cells can increase their visibility to immune cells and improve antigen presentation.
   - Approaches such as interferon gamma (IFN-γ) treatment or targeted therapies can upregulate HLA expression, making tumor cells more susceptible to immune recognition.

2. Tumor-Specific Antigen Targeting:

- Identifying and targeting tumor-specific antigens can enhance antigen recognition by immune cells.

- Personalized cancer vaccines or adoptive T cell therapies can be designed to target specific antigens expressed by the tumor, increasing the likelihood of immune recognition and response.

3. Combination with Targeted Therapies:

- Targeted therapies, such as tyrosine kinase inhibitors or inhibitors of oncogenic signaling pathways, can modulate the tumor microenvironment and improve antigen presentation.

- These therapies can reduce tumor burden, increase tumor cell visibility to immune cells, and enhance the overall immunogenicity of the tumor.

4. Peptide Vaccines:

- Peptide vaccines can be developed to deliver tumor-specific antigens to stimulate immune responses.

- These vaccines can enhance antigen presentation and recognition by providing specific tumor antigens to the immune system, promoting immune activation and antitumor responses.

5. Epigenetic Modulation:

- Alterations in epigenetic regulation can impact antigen presentation by tumor cells.

- Modulating DNA methylation or histone modifications can enhance the expression of genes involved in antigen presentation, improving the visibility of tumor cells to immune surveillance.

6. Tumor Cell Killing and Immunogenic Cell Death (ICD):

- Inducing immunogenic cell death of tumor cells can enhance antigen presentation.

- Certain treatments, such as radiation therapy or specific chemotherapeutic agents, can induce ICD, resulting in the release of tumor antigens and danger signals that promote immune recognition.

7. Co-Stimulatory Molecules and Adjuvants:

- Co-stimulatory molecules, such as CD40 or OX40 agonists, can enhance antigen presentation and immune activation.

- Adjuvants, such as Toll-like receptor agonists, can stimulate immune cells, promote antigen presentation, and improve immune responses.

8. Combination with Immune Checkpoint Inhibitors:

- Immune checkpoint inhibitors, such as PD-1/PD-L1 or CTLA-4 inhibitors, can restore T cell function and enhance antigen recognition.

- Combining immune checkpoint inhibitors with therapies aimed at improving antigen presentation can have synergistic effects, maximizing the antitumor immune response.

9. Biomarker-guided Therapy:

- Utilizing predictive biomarkers, such as tumor mutational burden or neoantigen profiling, can help identify patients who are more likely to respond to immunotherapy.

- Tailoring treatment strategies based on these biomarkers can optimize antigen presentation and recognition for individual patients.

Improving antigen presentation and recognition is a multifaceted approach that involves a combination of targeted therapies, vaccines, immunomodulators, and personalized treatment strategies. By enhancing the visibility of tumor antigens to the immune system, we can overcome resistance to immunotherapy and promote effective immune responses against cancer cells. Ongoing research and clinical trials are crucial for further understanding these strategies and optimizing their efficacy in different cancer types and patient populations.

ADVANCES IN PRECISION MEDICINE AND GENOMICS

Advances in precision medicine and genomics have significantly contributed to the development of new cancer immunotherapies, and ongoing research continues to shape the future of this field. Here are some future directions and potential advancements:

1. Personalized Immunotherapy:
   - Precision medicine aims to tailor treatments to individual patients based on their unique genetic and molecular characteristics.
   - Genomic profiling of tumors can identify specific alterations, such as neoantigens or immune-related gene expression patterns, that can guide the selection of immunotherapies.
   - Combining genomic information with immune profiling data can enable the identification of patients who are most likely to respond to specific immunotherapies, leading to more effective and personalized treatment strategies.

2. Neoantigen Vaccines:

- Neoantigens are tumor-specific antigens resulting from somatic mutations in cancer cells.

- Genomic sequencing and computational approaches can identify neoantigens, allowing for the design of personalized neoantigen vaccines.

- These vaccines can stimulate the immune system to specifically target and eliminate tumor cells, offering a highly personalized approach to cancer immunotherapy.

3. Combination Therapies:

- The future of cancer immunotherapy lies in the development of novel combination therapies.

- Genomic profiling can help identify specific molecular targets or signaling pathways that can be therapeutically exploited.

- Combining immunotherapies with targeted therapies, chemotherapy, radiation therapy, or other treatment modalities can enhance antitumor immune responses and overcome resistance mechanisms.

4. Biomarker Discovery:

- Continued advancements in genomics and other "-omics" technologies can lead to the discovery of novel biomarkers for immunotherapy response and resistance.

- Biomarkers, such as gene expression signatures, mutational burden, or immune cell infiltration patterns, can guide treatment decisions and help predict patient outcomes.

- Integration of multi-omics data, including genomics, transcriptomics, proteomics, and metabolomics, can provide a comprehensive understanding of the tumor-immune interaction and aid in the development of more effective immunotherapies.

5. Gene Editing and Cell Engineering:

- Gene editing technologies, such as CRISPR-Cas9, offer the potential to modify immune cells, making them more effective in targeting tumors.

- Genetic engineering can enhance the expression of specific receptors or signaling molecules on immune cells, improving their ability to recognize and kill cancer cells.

- Advances in cell engineering can also lead to the development of off-the-shelf, allogeneic cell therapies with enhanced tumor-targeting capabilities.

6. Microbiome and Immunotherapy:

- The gut microbiome has been linked to the efficacy of cancer immunotherapy.

- Understanding the interaction between the microbiome and the immune system can lead to the development of microbiome-based interventions to enhance immunotherapy outcomes.

- Modulating the microbiome through probiotics, fecal microbiota transplantation, or microbial metabolites may influence the response to immunotherapy and improve patient outcomes.

7. Artificial Intelligence (AI) and Machine Learning:

- AI and machine learning algorithms can process large-scale genomic and clinical data to identify patterns, predict treatment response, and uncover potential therapeutic targets.

- These technologies can aid in the development of precision immunotherapies by integrating multiple data sources, predicting patient outcomes, and optimizing treatment strategies.

8. Immune System Modeling and Simulation:

- Computational models that simulate the dynamics of the immune system can help predict and optimize immunotherapy outcomes.

- These models can simulate the interactions between immune cells, tumor cells, and therapeutic interventions, providing insights into treatment efficacy and identifying strategies to overcome resistance.

9. Liquid Biopsies:

- Liquid biopsies, such as circulating tumor DNA (ctDNA) analysis, can provide non-invasive and real

-time monitoring of tumor genetic alterations and immune responses.

- Liquid biopsies can help track treatment response, detect resistance mechanisms, and guide treatment adjustments in real-time, enabling timely modifications to immunotherapy strategies.

These future directions highlight the potential of precision medicine and genomics in advancing cancer immunotherapy. By harnessing the power of genomic information, personalized approaches, combination therapies, and innovative technologies, we can further improve treatment outcomes and overcome resistance, ultimately leading to better outcomes for patients with cancer. Continued research, collaboration, and clinical trials are key to translating these advancements into clinical practice.

FUTURE DIRECTIONS

The field of cancer immunotherapy is continually evolving, and several novel therapeutic targets and approaches are being explored to enhance the effectiveness of treatment. Here are some future directions in this area:

1. Next-generation Immune Checkpoint Inhibitors:

- While immune checkpoint inhibitors have shown remarkable success in some patients, not all individuals respond to these therapies.

- Future research aims to develop next-generation immune checkpoint inhibitors that target additional inhibitory molecules or pathways, providing broader and more potent immune activation.

2. Targeting Co-inhibitory Pathways:

- Beyond the well-known immune checkpoint molecules, there are other co-inhibitory pathways involved in immune regulation.

- Identifying and targeting these pathways, such as LAG-3, TIM-3, TIGIT, VISTA, or B7-H3, can potentially enhance T cell responses and overcome resistance.

3. Combination Immunotherapies:

- Combinations of different immunotherapies, such as immune checkpoint inhibitors, adoptive cell therapies, cancer vaccines, or cytokine therapies, are being explored to achieve synergistic effects and overcome resistance.

- Rational design and optimization of combination regimens based on preclinical and clinical data can lead to improved outcomes.

4. Genetically Engineered T cell Therapies:

- Advances in gene editing technologies, such as CRISPR-Cas9, are enabling precise modifications of T cells.

- Genetic engineering can enhance the specificity, functionality, and persistence of T cells, leading to improved tumor targeting and overall response rates.

5. Targeting Tumor Metabolism:

- Tumor cells often exhibit metabolic alterations that contribute to their survival and immune evasion.

- Targeting metabolic pathways, such as glycolysis, oxidative phosphorylation, or nutrient sensing, can impact tumor immune responses and improve the efficacy of immunotherapy.

6. Innate Immune Cell Activation:

- Besides T cells, innate immune cells, such

as natural killer (NK) cells or macrophages, play critical roles in antitumor immunity.

- Strategies to enhance the activation and cytotoxicity of these innate immune cells are being explored as potential immunotherapeutic approaches.

7. Microenvironment Modulation:

- The tumor microenvironment influences immune responses and can contribute to therapy resistance.

- Novel approaches aim to modulate the tumor microenvironment to promote immune cell infiltration, reduce immunosuppression, and enhance immunotherapy responses.

8. Combination with Other Treatment Modalities:

- Combining immunotherapy with conventional treatments, such as chemotherapy, radiation therapy, targeted therapies, or epigenetic modulators, can enhance treatment outcomes.

- Synergistic effects between immunotherapy and other modalities can lead to improved tumor control and long-term responses.

9. Development of Predictive Biomarkers:

- Identifying reliable predictive biomarkers can help select patients who are more likely to respond to specific immunotherapies.

- Research is focused on developing robust biomarkers, including genomic, immune, or molecular signatures, to guide treatment decisions and improve patient outcomes.

10. Artificial Intelligence and Machine Learning:

- The integration of AI and machine learning algorithms can aid in analyzing complex data sets, identifying patterns, and predicting treatment responses.

- AI-based tools can assist in treatment selection, patient stratification, and optimizing therapeutic combinations, ultimately leading to personalized immunotherapies.

These future directions hold great promise for advancing cancer immunotherapy and improving patient outcomes. Continued research, collaboration, and clinical trials are essential for translating these novel targets and approaches into clinical practice, ultimately benefiting a wider range of cancer patients.

MULTIDISCIPLINARY COLLABORATION AND CLINICAL TRIALS

Multidisciplinary collaboration and clinical trials play crucial roles in overcoming cancer immunotherapy resistance. Here are the key reasons why they are important:

1. Comprehensive Expertise:
   - Cancer immunotherapy resistance is a complex phenomenon influenced by various factors, including tumor biology, immune system interactions, and treatment modalities.
   - Multidisciplinary collaboration brings together experts from different fields, such as oncologists, immunologists, geneticists, pathologists, radiologists, and bioinformaticians.
   - The diverse expertise and perspectives fostered by collaboration enable a comprehensive understanding of the mechanisms underlying resistance and facilitate the development of effective strategies to overcome it.

2. Integration of Knowledge and Resources:

- Cancer immunotherapy resistance requires a multidimensional approach that integrates clinical observations, laboratory research, and technological advancements.

- Collaboration between clinicians and researchers allows for the translation of scientific discoveries into clinical applications.

- Clinical trials provide a platform to test new therapies, biomarkers, and treatment strategies in a controlled and rigorous manner, ensuring that findings are applicable to real-world patient care.

3. Identification of Biomarkers and Predictive Factors:

- Resistance mechanisms can be diverse and patient-specific, making it challenging to identify reliable biomarkers or predictive factors.

- Multidisciplinary collaboration allows for the pooling of diverse datasets, including genomic, proteomic, and clinical data, to identify robust biomarkers of resistance.

- Clinical trials provide the opportunity to validate these biomarkers and assess their predictive value in guiding treatment decisions.

4. Optimization of Treatment Strategies:

- Overcoming resistance often requires the development of innovative treatment strategies and therapeutic combinations.

- Multidisciplinary collaboration enables the

identification and evaluation of new targets, drugs, and treatment modalities that can be combined with immunotherapy.

- Clinical trials allow for the testing of these novel strategies in a systematic and controlled manner, providing evidence for their efficacy and safety.

5. Real-time Data Collection and Analysis:

- Multidisciplinary collaboration facilitates the collection and analysis of real-time clinical and scientific data.

- Regular interdisciplinary meetings and discussions allow for the timely exchange of information, enabling clinicians and researchers to adapt and modify treatment strategies based on emerging evidence.

- Clinical trials provide structured frameworks for data collection and analysis, ensuring high-quality and standardized data that can inform future treatment approaches.

6. Patient-Centric Approach:

- Multidisciplinary collaboration places the patient at the center of care, considering their individual characteristics, preferences, and needs.

- By bringing together experts from different disciplines, a personalized and tailored approach to overcoming resistance can be developed.

- Clinical trials provide opportunities for patients to access novel therapies, participate in research, and contribute to the advancement of cancer immunotherapy.

In summary, multidisciplinary collaboration and clinical trials are vital for understanding, addressing, and overcoming resistance to cancer immunotherapy. They foster comprehensive knowledge integration, facilitate the development and validation of biomarkers, optimize treatment strategies, and prioritize patient-centric care. Continued collaboration and participation in clinical trials are essential to drive progress in the field and improve outcomes for patients with resistant cancers.

CONCLUDING REMARKS

In conclusion, the ongoing efforts to overcome resistance to immunotherapy and improve cancer treatment outcomes are driven by the recognition of the complex nature of cancer and the dynamic interplay between tumors and the immune system. Researchers, clinicians, and scientists from various disciplines are collaborating to tackle the challenges associated with immunotherapy resistance, paving the way for more effective and personalized treatment strategies.

Through a deeper understanding of the mechanisms underlying resistance, innovative approaches are being developed to address the diverse factors contributing to treatment failure. Multidisciplinary collaboration has enabled the integration of knowledge and resources, leading to the identification of predictive biomarkers, the exploration of novel therapeutic targets, and the optimization of treatment combinations.

Clinical trials play a vital role in testing and validating these strategies, providing the evidence needed to guide clinical practice and improve patient outcomes. The continuous evaluation and refinement of treatment approaches based on real-time data and patient-specific characteristics allow for a more tailored and effective approach to cancer therapy.

Advancements in precision medicine, genomics, gene editing technologies, and the exploration of combination therapies offer new opportunities to enhance the effectiveness of immunotherapy. Additionally, efforts are being made to modulate the tumor microenvironment, improve T cell function, and optimize antigen presentation, recognizing the importance of both the tumor and the immune response in achieving durable responses.

The identification of resistance mechanisms, such as alterations in antigen presentation, upregulation of immune checkpoints, immune cell suppression, and tumor cell evolution, has provided valuable insights into potential targets for intervention. By targeting these mechanisms, we can overcome immunotherapy resistance and improve treatment outcomes.

While challenges remain, the collective efforts of the scientific community, healthcare professionals, and patients are driving progress in the field. Ongoing research, collaboration, and clinical trials are essential for translating these advancements into clinical practice, ensuring that more patients can benefit from the transformative potential of immunotherapy.

In conclusion, the pursuit of overcoming resistance to immunotherapy represents a promising frontier in cancer treatment. By combining scientific innovation, multidisciplinary collaboration, personalized approaches, and the integration of new technologies, we can improve cancer treatment outcomes and bring us closer to the goal of achieving long-lasting and curative responses for patients with cancer.

ABOUT THE AUTHOR

Dr. Bhratri Bhushan

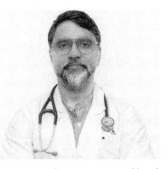

Dr. Bhratri Bhushan is a consultant medical oncologist and hematologist dedicated to the noble pursuit of healing and alleviating the suffering of his patients. His academic journey began at the renowned SMS Medical College in Jaipur, where he earned his MBBS degree, immersing himself in the profound knowledge of medicine. Fueled by a thirst for expertise, he pursued an MD in internal medicine at RNT Medical College in Udaipur.

Driven by an unwavering passion for oncology, he embarked on a super-specialization journey, delving into the captivating realm of medical oncology. This transformative phase of his education took place at the illustrious Gujarat Cancer and Research Institute & MP Shah Cancer

Hospital in Ahmedabad, one of the largest cancer institutes in Asia. Under the guidance of the institute, he received comprehensive training in medical oncology, hematology, pediatric oncology, bone marrow transplantation, and the compassionate field of palliative medicine.

Presently, he has the privilege of serving as a consultant medical oncologist and hematologist at the esteemed Ananta Institute of Medical Sciences and Research Centre. In this role, he contributes as a Professor of Medicine, imparting knowledge and guiding the next generation of medical professionals. Prior to this, he held a prominent position as a consultant and Head of the Department of Medical Oncology at Jindal Institute of Medical Sciences in Hisar.

Over the course of his career, he has had the honour of administering over 50,000 chemotherapy cycles to patients battling cancer. At their state-of-the-art center, they have meticulously crafted a sanctuary for healing, equipped with cutting-edge facilities. The arsenal includes the remarkable Varian linear accelerator for delivering precise radiation therapy, PET-CT scan, Gamma camera, and a modular operation theatre adorned with laparoscopy compatibility, enabling him to perform a diverse range of cancer surgeries. At their center, they also provides hyperthermic intraperitoneal chemotherapy for those confronting advanced stages of cancer. Their dedicated chemotherapy daycare ward, equipped with biosafety cabinets, offers a sanctuary of comfort and care. Furthermore, they offer a comprehensive array of cancer medicines, ranging from conventional cytotoxic chemotherapy to targeted therapy, immunotherapy, hormonal therapy, palliative medicines, pain management services, and rehabilitation services.

With unwavering dedication, his esteemed team and he treat an extensive spectrum of cancers, encompassing solid malignancies, hematological malignancies, benign hematology conditions, gynecological cancers, and pediatric cancers. Their mission is rooted in the pursuit of providing exceptional quality care at an affordable cost, ensuring that their patients receive the utmost attention and compassionate support.

The culmination of his relentless pursuit of excellence has garnered recognition and accolades from esteemed institutions and organizations. He has been bestowed with prestigious awards such as the Rajasthan Gaurav Award, Bharat Jyoti Award, Rastriya Chikitsa Ratan Award, Asia's Top Doctor Award, Healthcare Excellence Award by Brands Impact, Excellence in Oncology Indian Health Professional Award, National Education Brilliance Award, Education Leadership Award,

International Leadership Award, and many more. These accolades stand as a testament to his unwavering commitment to his profession and his tireless efforts to advance the field of oncology.

Beyond his contributions to academia, he has also made significant literary contributions. His publications transcend the boundaries of medicine, with more than 150 books on the subject of oncology and medicine, many of which have achieved the coveted status of bestsellers. In esteemed international journals, his voice resonates through articles, reviews, case studies, and research papers, sharing invaluable insights with his peers. However, his creative spirit finds solace in the realm of poetry. He has poured his heart and soul into crafting many poetry books, each containing his internationally acclaimed and award-winning verses.

Among his literary achievements, some of his bestselling books have become cherished companions for patients navigating the challenges of various kinds of cancers. These survival guides serve as beacons of hope, offering solace, guidance, and empowering knowledge to those on their arduous journeys. In addition, his works encompass a comprehensive review of all kinds of cancers for oncologists and other medical professionals.